O R M

OXFORD RESPIRATORY MEDICINE LIBRARY

Cystic Fibrosis

Second Edition

O R M L

OXFORD RESPIRATORY MEDICINE LIBRARY

Cystic Fibrosis

Second Edition

Edited by

Dr Alex Horsley

Senior Lecturer and Honorary Consultant, University of Manchester,
Manchester Adult Cystic Fibrosis Centre,
University Hospital of South Manchester,
Wythenshawe Hospital,
Manchester, UK

Dr Steve Cunningham

Consultant Respiratory Paediatrician and Honorary Reader,
Department of Child Health and Life,
Royal Hospital for Sick Children,
Edinburgh, UK

Dr J Alastair Innes

Consultant Physician and Honorary Reader in Respiratory Medicine,
Scottish Adult CF Service,
Western General Hospital,
Edinburgh, UK

OXFORD
UNIVERSITY PRESS

OXFORD
UNIVERSITY PRESS

Great Clarendon Street, Oxford, OX2 6DP,
United Kingdom

Oxford University Press is a department of the University of Oxford.
It furthers the University's objective of excellence in research, scholarship,
and education by publishing worldwide. Oxford is a registered trade mark of
Oxford University Press in the UK and in certain other countries

© Oxford University Press 2015

The moral rights of the authors have been asserted

First Edition published in 2010
Second edition published in 2015

Impression: 1

Published in the United States of America by Oxford University Press
198 Madison Avenue, New York, NY 10016, United States of America

British Library Cataloguing in Publication Data:

Data available

Library of Congress Control Number:

Data available

ISBN 978–0–19–870294–8

Printed and bound in Great Britain by
Clays Ltd, St Ives plc

Contents

Foreword

The progress made in the treatment of people with cystic fibrosis (CF) over the past four decades has been one of medicine's success stories. The delivery of clinical expertise by multidisciplinary teams combined with innovative approaches to antibiotic therapy and mucus clearance have increased the quality of life of people with CF and significantly increased their survival. In the past five years drugs which correct the function of the CFTR protein have demonstrated that a transformative clinical impact can result from an understanding and treatment of the basic defect. Disease modifying therapies based on a stratified medicine approach to different classes of mutation are likely to become routine therapy for people with CF over the next 5 years.

The outlook for people with CF is now considerably more positive compared to 20 years ago with current median survival of greater than 40 years in most developed countries, a result of CF centre care and effective treatment of infection. This has resulted in a steady increase in the number of people with CF, particularly those at adult age, which is likely to increase further with innovative new treatments modulating the basic defect. In most developed countries adults now outnumber children with CF, and by 2025 it is estimated that there will be a further 100% increase in the number of adults.

The pulmonary and systemic morbidities of CF, however, have not gone away despite these treatment advances. It is critically important that optimal therapy is delivered by multidisciplinary teams to maintain lung health and treat the other multisystem complications of this condition. Treating CF is complicated and challenges clinicians at all levels to think hard about diagnoses, diagnostics, and treatment. This all has to be considered in people with life ambitions such as family, education, and career. This edition of Cystic Fibrosis is very timely as it provides a state-of-the-art summary of the underlying pathophysiology and the important diagnostics and treatments of this condition. This book is comprehensive and detailed in the important areas of care delivery and provides an excellent introduction and practical support manual for clinical trainees from a range of disciplines who deliver care for patients with CF. This book is mandatory reading for all trainees in respiratory medicine and, increasingly, in general internal medicine as the number of people with CF attending clinics with complications in other organ systems is increasing. It will also be a must-have reference for the multidisciplinary teams providing CF centre care. I believe this will also inspire medical students undertaking placements or modules in CF to widen their understanding of the disease and hopefully inspire them to commit to careers in providing care for people with this devastating disease.

The editors and authors are to be commended for producing an up-to-date, relevant, and practical short textbook to help multidisciplinary teams manage their patients better. Tools such as this will help us to further improve CF care across the world.

J Stuart Elborn
President of the European Cystic Fibrosis Society, and
Dean of Medicine, Dentistry and Biomedical Sciences
Queens University Belfast
23 January 2015

Preface

The treatment of cystic fibrosis (CF), and the outlook for patients, is one of the major successes of modern translational medicine. Understanding of the genetics of the disease has led to widespread newborn screening, so that the diagnosis is made early before lung damage is evident. Knowledge of the pathophysiology of lung disease has led to advances in the treatment of lung infections and inflammation, with continuing improvements in survival and morbidity. CF has become a chronic disease of adulthood rather than an acute disease of children.

We have now entered a new phase of disease management, characterized by CF-mutation-specific therapies that for the first time address the basic defect in CF rather than merely the consequences. Not since the CF gene was isolated over a quarter of a century ago has there been such excitement in the field of CF care. On the other hand, many challenges remain. As patients live longer, new problems and challenges are being faced and the treatment burden for patients continues to grow. Despite being a single gene disorder, a genetic cure remains elusive.

Pulmonary infections and progressive respiratory failure are the primary causes of mortality and morbidity, and patients are usually cared for by respiratory specialist teams. CF, however, is a multi-system disease, and the treatment and management of patients with CF necessarily involves many different specialists, from different disciplines of medicine and associated professions. With increased survival, management of these other complications becomes more relevant, and it is clear that earlier recognition and treatment of non-respiratory complications will form an important part of future CF care. In this second edition, these sections have continued to expand as our knowledge of the complications, and the options for treatment, increase. This book is aimed at all involved in the care of CF patients and we hope that we have succeeded in covering the broad range of problems faced by the both adult and paediatric teams.

Much of the management of patients with CF is based upon what is thought to be best practice, rather than large randomized controlled trials. There is thus bound to be some variation in practice between different units and countries. Where suggestions have been made, in the absence of unequivocal evidence, they remain just that, and may differ from local policy. We hope, however, that where guidance has been offered that it will prove useful, even if not identical to local practice.

Alex Horsley
Manchester 2015

Contributors

Jane Ashbrook

Advanced Musculoskeletal Physiotherapist
Manchester Adult Cystic Fibrosis Centre
University Hospital of South Manchester
Manchester, UK

John Blaikley

Senior Lecturer and Honorary Consultant
    Physician
Lung Transplant Centre
University Hospital of South Manchester
Manchester, UK

Sally Connolly

Consultant Paediatrician
Sheffield Children's Hospital
Sheffield, UK

Katrina Cox

Specialist Cystic Fibrosis Pharmacist
Manchester Adult Cystic Fibrosis Centre
University Hospital of South Manchester
Manchester, UK

Steve Cunningham

Consultant Respiratory Paediatrician &
    Senior Lecturer
Department of Child Life & Health
Royal Hospital for Sick Children
Edinburgh, UK

Jane C Davies

Professor & Honorary Consultant in
    Paediatric Respiratory Medicine
Royal Brompton and Harefield NHS Trust
Imperial College, London, UK

Elaine Dhouieb

Physiotherapy Respiratory
    Clinical Lead
Royal Hospital for Sick Children
Edinburgh, UK

Alistair JA Duff

Head of Psychology Services & Consultant
    Clinical Psychologist
Honorary Clinical Associate Professor
School of Medicine, University of Leeds, UK

Frank P Edenborough

Consultant Respiratory Physician
Sheffield Adult Cystic Fibrosis Centre
Sheffield, UK

Rosanna Featherstone

Paediatric Research Nurse
Department of Gene Therapy
National Heart and Lung Institute
Imperial College, London, UK

Andrew J Fisher

Professor of Respiratory Transplant
    Medicine & Honorary Consultant Chest
    Physician
Institute of Transplantation
Freeman Hospital
Newcastle Upon Tyne, UK

Francis J Gilchrist

Lecturer and Consultant in Paediatric
    Respiratory Medicine
University Hospital of North Staffordshire
Stoke on Trent, UK

John Govan

Professor Emeritus in Microbial
    Pathogenicity
University of Edinburgh Medical School
Edinburgh, UK

Charles Haworth

Consultant Respiratory Physician
Cambridge Centre for Lung Infection
Papworth Hospital
Cambridge, UK

Uta Hill

Consultant Respiratory Physician
Cambridge Centre for Lung Infection
Papworth Hospital
Cambridge, UK

Alex Horsley

Senior Lecturer & Honorary Consultant
University of Manchester
Manchester Adult Cystic Fibrosis Centre
University Hospital of South Manchester
Manchester, UK

J Alastair Innes

Consultant Physician & Honorary Reader in
    Respiratory Medicine
Scottish Adult CF Service
Western General Hospital
Edinburgh, UK

Andrew Jones

Consultant Physician & Honorary Reader in
    Respiratory Medicine
Manchester Adult Cystic Fibrosis Centre
University Hospital of South Manchester
Manchester, UK

Antoinette Moran

Division Chief & Professor of Paediatric
    Endocrinology
University of Minnesota
Minneapolis, USA

Stephen MP O'Riordan

Consultant in Paediatric Endocrinology &
    Diabetes
Honorary Senior Lecturer
University College Cork
Cork, Ireland

Chris Orchard

Cystic Fibrosis Research Fellow
Department of Cystic Fibrosis
Royal Brompton Hospital and Imperial
    College
London, UK

Helen Oxley

Consultant Clinical Psychologist
Manchester Adult Cystic Fibrosis Centre
Wythenshawe Hospital
Manchester, UK

Nicholas Simmonds

Consultant Respiratory Physician &
    Honorary Senior Lecturer
Department of Cystic Fibrosis
Royal Brompton Hospital and Imperial
    College
London, UK

Christopher Taylor

Professor of Paediatric Gastroenterology
Academic Unit of Child Health
University of Sheffield
Sheffield, UK

Rebecca Thursfield

Paediatric Respiratory Research Fellow
Department of Respiratory Paediatrics
Royal Brompton Hospital and Imperial
    College
London, UK

Abbreviations

ABPA	allergic bronchopulmonary aspergillosis
ACBT	active cycle of breathing technique
ACT	airway clearance techniques
AD	autogenic drainage
ADD	adaptive aerosol delivery
ARFI	acoustic-radiation-force impulse
ART	assisted reproductive techniques
BAL	bronchoalveolar lavage
BCC	*Burkholderia cepacia* complex
BD	twice daily
BG	blood glucose
BMD	bone mineral density
BMI	body mass index
BNF	British National Formulary
BOS	*Bronchiolitis obliterans syndrome*
BPFAS	Behavioral Pediatric Feeding Assessment Scale
CBAVD	congenital bilateral absence of the *vas deferens*
CBT	cognitive behaviour therapy
CF	cystic fibrosis
CFA	cystic fibrosis-related arthropathy
CFQ	Cystic Fibrosis Questionnaire
CFSPID	CF screen positive, inconclusive diagnosis
CLAD	chronic lung allograft dysfunction
CFRD	CF-related diabetes
CFRD FH-	CF-related diabetes without fasting hyperglycemia
CFRD FH+	CF-related diabetes with fasting hyperglycemia
CFTR	cystic fibrosis transmembrane conductance regulator
CGM	continuous glucose monitoring
CMV	Cytomegalovirus
CT	computed tomography
DIOS	distal ileal obstruction syndrome
DMARD	disease-modifying anti-rheumatic drugs
DXA	dual-energy X-ray absorptiometry
EBV	Epstein–Barr virus

ECMO	extracorporeal membrane oxygenation
ENaC	epithelial sodium channel
EPAP	expiratory positive airway pressure
ERCF	European Epidemiologic Registry of Cystic Fibrosis
EVLP	ex-vivo lung perfusion
FEV$_1$	forced expiratory volume in 1 second
FRC	functional residual capacity
FSH	follicle-stimulating hormone
FTI	fosfomycin in combination with tobramycin
GORD	gastro-oesophageal reflux disease
HCG	human chorionic gonadotrophin
HFCWO	high frequency chest wall oscillation
HIVAT	home intravenous antibiotic treatment
HRTC	high-resolution computed tomography
IAPP	islet amyloid polypeptide
IGT	impaired glucose tolerance
HOA	hypertrophic osteoarthropathy
HS	hypertonic saline
IBAT	ileal bile acid transporter
ICSI	intracytcoplasmic sperm injection
IGT	impaired glucose tolerance
IPAP	inspiratory positive airway pressure
IPV	intrapulmonary percussive vibration
IRT	immune reactive trypsin
IUD	intrauterine device
IUI	intrauterine sperm injection
IVF	in vitro fertilization
LCI	lung clearance index
MBL	Mannose-binding lectin
MI	Meconium ileus
MRSA	meticillin-resistant S. aureus
NG	nastrogastric
NGT	normal glucose tolerance
NIV	non-invasive ventilation
NPD	nasal potential difference
NTM	non-tuberculous mycobacteria
OB	obliterative bronchiolitis
OD	once daily
OGTT	oral glucose tolerance testing
OPEP	intrathoracic oscillating positive expiratory pressure

Pa	*Pseudomonas aeruginosa*
PCL	pericilliary layer
PEG	percutaneous endoscopic gastrostomy
PEP	positive expiratory pressure
PERT	pancreatic enzyme replacement therapy
PESA	percutaneous epididymal sperm aspiration
PGD	pre-implantation genetic diagnosis
PI	pancreatic insufficiency
PICC	peripherally inserted central catheters
PRN	when required
PTC	premature termination codon
PTLD	*post-transplant lymphoproliferative disorder*
PTH	parathyroid hormone
PVL	Panton–Valentine leukocidin
QDS	four times daily
QoL	quality of life
QS	quorum sensing
RAS	restrictive allograft syndrome
T1D	type 1 diabetes
T2D	type 2 diabetes
TDS	three times daily
TESA	testicular sperm aspiration
TESE	testicular sperm extraction
TIPPS	transjugular intra-hepatic portosystemic shunting
TIVAD	totally implantable venous access device
TLC	total lung capacity
UI	urinary incontinence
VMT	vibrating mesh technology

Chapter 1

Genetics and pathophysiology

Alex Horsley

'The child will soon die whose forehead tastes salty when kissed'
(Almanac of Children's Songs and Games, Switzerland 1857)

Key points

- Cystic fibrosis (CF) is the most common autosomal recessive disease in Caucasians associated with early death
- Unaffected carrier frequency is 1:25
- ΔF508 (Phe508del) is the most common of over 1900 mutations
- The gene encodes a transmembrane chloride conductance channel, the CFTR, which regulates chloride ion and water movements across the cell membrane
- CFTR is expressed throughout the body, and CF disease affects multiple systems, including major effects on the lung, pancreas, and gastrointestinal systems
- Pulmonary disease is the most important cause of death and disability, resulting from chronic progressive suppurative lung disease
- Over-activation of the sodium (ENaC) channel in the lungs, caused by loss of CFTR-inhibition, results in dehydration of the airway surface fluid layer and consequent poor mucociliary clearance
- Retained secretions encourage bacterial adherence, chronic neutrophillic inflammation, and a vicious cycle of infection, inflammation, and tissue destruction

1.1 Introduction

Cystic fibrosis (CF) is a complex multisystem disease, caused by defects in a single gene. Pulmonary manifestations are responsible for most of the morbidity and mortality, and the hallmark of the condition is progressive and irreversible bronchiectasis and respiratory failure. However, the condition also has important effects on gastrointestinal function, nutrition, endocrine, metabolic, and reproductive systems.

1.2 Inheritance

Cystic fibrosis is the most common life-shortening genetic disorder of those of Western European origin. The faulty gene, on the long arm of chromosome 7, was identified in 1989. It encodes an epithelial ion channel known as the cystic fibrosis transmembrane conductance regulator (CFTR). Carriers of a single faulty gene are asymptomatic and CF is caused by co-inheritance of two disease-causing mutant alleles of the CFTR gene, one from each parent

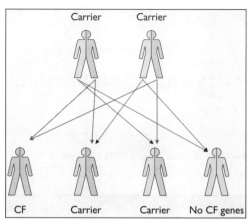

Figure 1.1 Inheritance of CF. Each parent carries a single copy of a defective CF gene, but because they have one normal copy they are asymptomatic. There is a 1:4 chance of producing a CF child, and half of all their children will also be carriers.

(Figure 1.1). The condition has a carrier frequency of 1:25 in those of European descent and affects 1 in 2500–3000 live births in the UK and Western Europe. This high incidence may be explained by a possible protective effect in CF carriers against gastrointestinal infections such as typhoid or cholera.

Over 1900 CFTR mutations have been described, although many of these do not cause disease. The most common CF mutation is a deletion of three base pairs (CTT) encoding phenylalanine at position 508, known as Phe508del because of its effect on the CFTR protein (Phe = phenylalanine, del = deletion), ΔF508 (Δ = 'delta', or deletion, and F = phenylalanine) or F508del. This is largely responsible for the high incidence of CF in the Caucasian population, where it accounts for over two-thirds of CF mutations. Many patients will be compound heterozygotes, containing one copy of the ΔF508 gene and one other mutation.

1.3 Cystic fibrosis transmembrane regulator

1.3.1 Structure and function of CFTR

The protein encoded by the CFTR gene comprises 1480 amino acids. CFTR is a member of a class of proteins termed the ATP-binding cassette (ABC) family. The protein spans cell membranes at two adjacent points to form a central channel (Figure 1.2). CFTR protein also has two nucleotide binding domains (NBD 1 and 2), which are capable of opening and closing the channel by hydrolysis of ATP. CFTR functions as a channel for chloride and (to a lesser extent) bicarbonate ions, and ion flow is regulated by protein kinase A.

CFTR in sweat glands is normally responsible for chloride, and hence sodium, reabsorption. It is the failure of this mechanism in CF that leads to excessive excretion of salt, and the salty taste described in the Swiss nursery rhyme quoted at the start of the chapter. This also forms the basis of the sweat test for diagnosis of CF (see Chapter 2).

The ΔF508 mutation occurs on NBD1 and prevents normal folding into the appropriate tertiary structure, resulting in cellular retention and degradation (a class II mutation, see section 1.4).

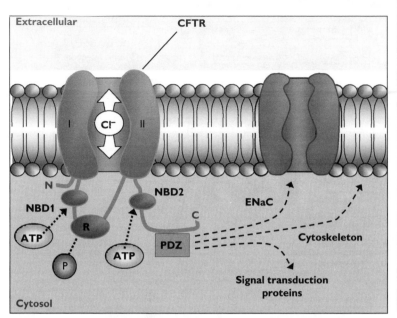

Figure 1.2 Structure of CFTR. The protein is expressed in apical cell membranes where it functions as a chloride channel. The channel is made up of two membrane spanning domains (I and II), each consisting of 6 membrane-spanning alpha helices. Two nucleotide binding domains (NBD1 and NBD2) mediate ATP hydrolysis, and it is on one of these (NBD1) that the most common CFTR mutation (ΔF508) occurs. Phosphorylation of the R domain permits a conformational change and opening of the channel. CFTR interacts through its C terminus with an array of different cellular proteins, including cytoskeleton, cell signaling mechanisms, and other ion channels, in particular the epithelial sodium channel ENaC.

1.3.2 **Interaction with other proteins**

CFTR forms part of a multi-protein assembly in the apical plasma membrane, and is involved in the regulation of a number of cellular processes. In particular it acts to down-regulate the activity of the transepithelial sodium channel (ENaC) in the apical epithelial membrane, an interaction with important consequences for the effects in the lung. In addition to this, it also interacts with calcium-activated chloride channels, potassium channels, sodium-bicarbonate transporters, and aquaporin water channels. Variability in the function of these other proteins are potential modifiers of the CF phenotype. CFTR is also able to form dimers in the plasma membrane, which may act to increase channel activity and/or reduce endocytic retrieval of CFTR from the membrane.

1.4 **Pathophysiology**

CFTR is expressed in epithelia throughout the body, and affects exocrine (secretory) function in a number of organs, including the lung, liver, gut, pancreas, and sweat glands. Most of the epithelial sites of expression correspond well with the known clinical effects of CF (Figure 1.3). The extra-pulmonary effects of CF will be described in the individual chapters dealing with these organs. The pulmonary manifestations, however, are the most important in terms of the burden of disease and survival.

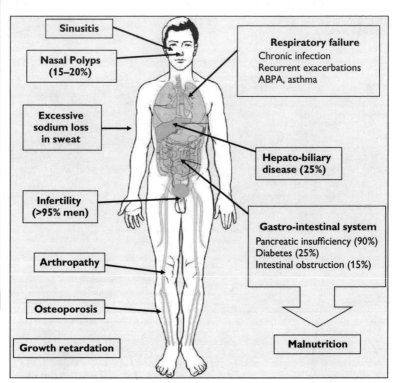

Figure 1.3 Clinical consequences of CF. Percentages in brackets represent the approximate percentages of CF patients affected in this way.

1.4.1 Lung disease in cystic fibrosis

In the lung, CFTR is detectable on the apical membrane of ciliated cells within the gland ducts and in the superficial epithelium of healthy individuals. In CF, the submucosal glands and distal airways are obstructed by thick tenacious secretions, resulting in a failure of normal mucociliary clearance and defective airway defence mechanisms against bacterial infection.

Low volume hypothesis

The most widely accepted explanation for the clinical effects of CFTR deficiency in the lung is known as the low volume hypothesis (see Figure 1.4). This proposes that, since CFTR normally functions to down-regulate ENaC, loss of CFTR function leads to over-activity of ENaC. Excessive Na^+ is therefore absorbed, and Cl^- follows through non-CFTR Cl^- channels. Mouse models with defective CFTR do not exhibit the classic pulmonary features of CF, whereas a mouse model with excessive ENaC activity has a lung phenotype similar to that of human CF. This leads to net absorption of ions and fluid, with consequent shrinking of airway surface liquid and dehydration of mucus secretions. The effects of this on the mucus layer and the cilia are crucial in the development of CF lung disease.

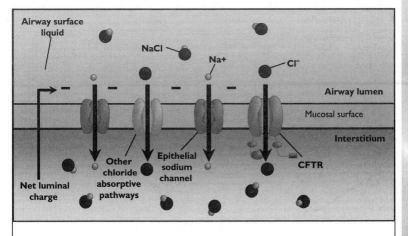

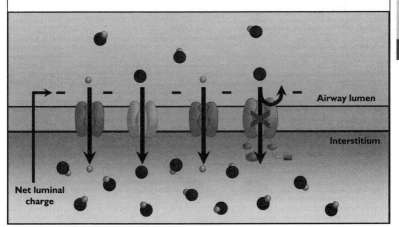

Figure 1.4 Low volume hypothesis for pathophysiology of CF in airway epithelium. In the normal situation (top), CFTR absorbs chloride ions (Cl^-), and regulates absorption of sodium (Na^+) through ENaC channels. In CF (bottom), inhibition of ENaC is abolished, leading to hyper-absorption of Na^+. Cl^- follows through alternative Cl^- channels, and water follows this, leading to shrinkage of the airway surface liquid and hyperpolarization of the epithelial surface.

Effects on mucus clearance

In health, the mucus layer is a gel consisting of around 1% salt, 1% high molecular weight secreted mucins, and 98% water. At its inner surface, between the mucus layer and the epithelial cell membrane, lies a thin pericilliary liquid layer. This layer provides a low viscosity solution in which the cilia can beat rapidly. It also prevents adhesion of the mucus to the epithelial surface, thereby lubricating the movement of mucus during cough clearance. Healthy airway epithelia in culture maintain an airway surface liquid (ASL) depth of 7μm, but CF airway epithelia continue to absorb the ASL and the cilia collapse onto the cell surface.

Unregulated absorption of ions and water across the CF airway epithelium causes shrinkage of the pericilliary liquid layer in CF and dehydration of the overlying mucus layer (Figure 1.5).

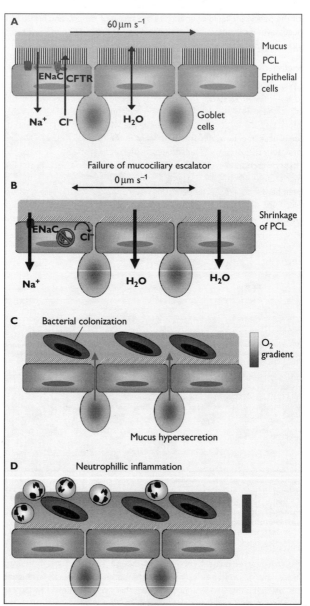

Figure 1.5 Proposed mechanism for the development of chronic airway infection in CF, after Boucher (2007). In normal airways (A), hydration is controlled by Na+ absorption and Cl- secretion. In CF (B), the absence of CFTR leads to unregulated Na+ absorption and associated dehydration of the pericilliary layer (PCL) and mucus. Mucus becomes adherent in plaques which allow bacterial colonization (C), encouraged by a hypoxic gradient across the plaque. The resulting inflammatory response (D) leads to a vicious cycle of inflammation, mucus secretion and retention, and ultimately airway destruction.

Data from the *Annual Review of Medicine*, Volume 58, ©2007 by Annual Reviews <http:www.annualreviews.org>

Shrinkage of the pericilliary liquid layer impairs the action of the cilia and brings an increasingly adhesive mucus layer into contact with the epithelium. The disruption of mucociliary clearance leads to mucus plugging which causes airway obstruction and promotes bacterial infection.

Vicious cycle of infection and inflammation

The exact process by which infection occurs is unclear but may comprise inhaled bacteria that are not cleared efficiently or the initial infection may follow an insult to the lung, e.g. viral infection or aspiration. Whatever the initiating event, lungs of CF patients often become colonized early in the course of the disease with bacteria such as Staphylococci or *H. influenzae*. These infections become persistent in the first few years of life and there is a florid inflammatory response that leads to neutrophil recruitment and activation. This in turn stimulates hypersecretion of mucin. Bacterial products and cellular debris accumulate, along with polymeric DNA (from bacteria and neutrophils) which makes the mucus more viscous and even harder to expel. The persisting neutrophil-dominated inflammatory response leads to release of neutrophil proteases, such as elastase and matrix metallo-proteinases. These cause proteolysis and chondrolysis of airway support tissue, with consequent airway dilatation and bronchiectasis. The CF airways fill up with purulent secretions and a vicious cycle of infection, inflammation, and progressive endobronchial destruction is established (Figure 1.6).

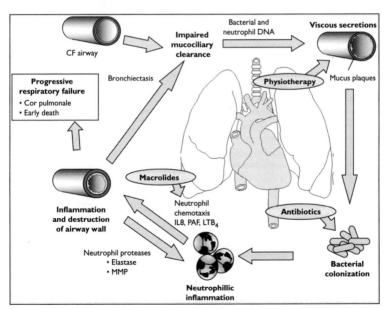

Figure 1.6 Vicious cycle of infection and inflammation in CF airways. Impaired mucociliary clearance in CF leads to retention of mucus, allowing bacterial colonization and subsequent neutrophillic inflammation. This results in mucosal and airway wall damage, progressing to bronchiectasis and ultimately to respiratory failure. Goblet cell hyperplasia results in increased mucus secretion, in turn made more viscous by release of cellular and bacterial DNA. Therapeutic interventions are shown in blue ovals, with the proposed site of action indicated.

1.4.2 **Clinical course**

The manifestations of CF lung disease are highly variable in onset and intensity. The clinical course is typically punctuated by periods of exacerbation, when bacterial infection gains the upper hand over host defence. At these times there is usually deterioration in lung function, and associated symptoms of infection (see Chapter 5). Some organisms, particularly *Pseudomonas aeruginosa* and *Burkholderia cepacia* (see Chapter 3), are associated with greater inflammation.

Chronic Pseudomonas infection

Pseudomonas aeruginosa is an important opportunistic infection in CF, and becomes established in the majority of patients by their late teens. It exists in two forms, a non-mucoid form and a mucoid form that, once established, is resistant to eradication (see Chapter 3). The formation of mucoid *Pseudomonas* biofilms appears to be encouraged by the thickened mucus in the CF airways. Mucus limits bacterial motility and diffusion of excreted proteins and the resulting high bacterial densities are detected by the bacteria's quorum-sensing mechanisms, which triggers a phenotypic change to biofilm forms. In addition, the thick mucus layer and the increased oxygen consumption of the epithelial cells leads to an oxygen gradient across the mucus, with particularly hypoxic areas in mucus plugs. This hypoxic environment favours the growth of *Pseudomonas* and switching to biofilm formation (Figure 1.5).

1.4.3 **CFTR and the immune system**

Impaired mucociliary clearance may not be the only significant process occurring in the CF lung. Other diseases are also associated with failure of mucociliary clearance, in particular primary ciliary dyskinesia, which has bronchiectasis as a common clinical feature, but generally has a far greater life expectancy than is seen in CF.

In patients with CF, a number of studies of infant bronchoalveolar lavage (BAL) fluid have found evidence of airway inflammation without concurrent lower airway infection. It may be that defective CFTR leads to dysregulation of the host defences in other more complex ways.

The innate defences of the airways consist of three main components, and there is evidence for deficiency in all three of these in CF (Figure 1.7). Impairment of the physical defence provided by the mucociliary escalator is described earlier in this chapter, and is certainly a major component of the lung pathophysiology in CF. There may also be impairment in the humoral defences, including defensins, antioxidants such as glutathione S transferase, and surfactant proteins. Finally, there is increasing evidence for impairments in cell-mediated immunity. CFTR is involved in lysosomal acidification via the counter-effect of Cl^- on H^+ accumulation, and this may be deficient in CF. CF neutrophils also appear to have an exaggerated response to inflammatory stimuli, associated with a reduced ability to phagocytose and clear bacteria. It is likely that a combination of these different mechanisms is responsible for the sustained inflammation that is the hallmark of CF pulmonary disease.

1.5 **CFTR gene mutations**

CF mutations vary in how they affect CFTR function. Those mutations leaving little functioning CFTR have most significant clinical effect, whereas those mutations leaving some residual CFTR function have fewer clinical effects. Milder mutations in compound heterozygotes have a dominant effect (i.e. a severe and a mild mutation combined will usually have mild disease).

1.5.1 **Class of mutation**

CF mutations are grouped into six classes depending on their effect on gene expression and CFTR function (see Figure 1.8).

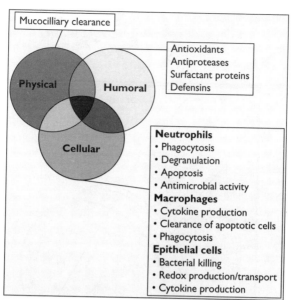

Figure 1.7 Effects of CF on innate immune system. Lung disease in CF is a consequence not purely of dysfunctional mucociliary clearance but also impairments in humoral and cellular immunity. The final phenotype is a consequence of the interaction between all of these factors.

- Class I: Transcription errors resulting in unstable, truncated, or no protein expression
- Class II: Defective protein maturation and trafficking. ΔF508 is an example of this sort of mutation
- Class III: Impaired chloride channel activity, primarily due to defects in the two NBDs
- Class IV: Defective channel gating and reduced chloride conductance
- Class V: Splicing abnormalities resulting in reduced amounts of functional protein
- Class VI: Accelerated turnover

The class of mutation that individual patients possess has recently become a far more important issue than previously. Ivacaftor is the first of a new category of orally available drugs that acts directly on the CFTR to increase the open probability of the chloride channel, leading to partial correction of the sweat chloride defect and impressive improvement in clinical parameters (see Chapters 3 and 13). The drug requires CFTR to be present at the cell surface in order to be effective (class III and IV mutations). Although the drug is licensed only for those with the class III mutation G551D at time of writing, this mainly reflects that this is the only individual mutation common enough for trials to be conducted on it. *In vitro*, the drug shows activity against a much broader range of class III and IV mutations, including the relatively common class IV mutation R117H. As more data become available, access to this expensive but effective drug is likely to be expanded.

1.5.2 Relationship between genotype and phenotype

Clinical severity is broadly related to the amount of residual CFTR activity. At one end of the spectrum (class I and II), little or no CFTR activity gives rise to severe lung disease. With

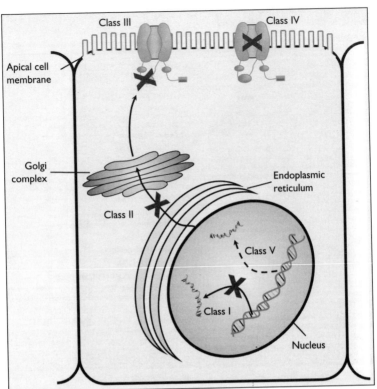

Figure 1.8 Classes of CFTR mutation and their effect on gene expression. Class I mutation—transcription errors; Class II—defective protein maturation and trafficking; Class III—impaired chloride channel activity; Class IV—defective channel gating; Class V—splicing abnormalities. The first two of these are associated with particularly diminished or absent CFTR activity and more severe clinical phenotypes.

Adapted from Rowe, et al. (2005).

increasing levels of residual CFTR function (class III, IV, V), pancreatic sufficiency is maintained, which has important prognostic implications. For instance, the presence of the class IV mutation R117H is reliably associated with pancreatic sufficiency. Just under 5% of the healthy CFTR mRNA levels appear to be sufficient to prevent the development of severe lung disease. Class V mutations may be associated with particularly mild phenotypes (e.g. congenital bilateral absence of vas deferens, with no other clinical manifestations of CF).

A list of common mutations, and their clinical effects, is given in Table 1.1. There are distinct differences in allele frequencies between the Caucasian population and those of different ethnic background, which has implications for screening. CF is much rarer in those of Asian descent than in Caucasians, but it may also be missed if only a limited genetic screen for common mutations is applied. The CF-EU2 assay used in the UK screens for the 50 most common CF mutations, and in accounts for 93% of mutations in patients of white British origin. The same panel however will only detect 21% of mutations in those of Pakistani origin, and a CF–Asian panel of mutations is used to screen these patients. Regardless of ethnic origins, discussion with the genetic laboratory and full exon sequencing may be required if clinical suspicion is high.

Table 1.1 Frequency of common CFTR mutations in the UK

Mutation	Class	Frequency (% CFTR)	Notes
ΔF508	II	90.7	Most common CF mutation
G551D	III	5.6	Associated with lower frequency of meconium ileus and later age of PI. Corrected with ivacaftor (Chapt. 3).
R117H	IV	4.3	Mild mutation, more severe when inherited in cis with the 5T variant of the poly-T tract. 7T results in mild disease. May be associated with preserved pancreatic function, minimal or no respiratory symptoms and CBAVD.
G542X	I	3.6	More common in patients of Asian* origin (frequency 25.6%)
621+1G→T	I	2.1	
N1303K	II	1.3	
1717-1G>A	I	1.3	
DI507	II	1.0	
R560T	III	1.0	
3659delC	II	1.0	
R553X	I	0.8	
3849+10kb→T	V	0.9	Associated with preserved pancreatic function.
Y569D	III	<0.1	Common in UK Pakistani popn. (frequency 9.6%)

*Asian refers to those of Pakistani, Indian, Bangladeshi, and other Asian descent.
CBAVD: Congenital bilateral absence of the vas deferens (male infertility).
PI: Pancreatic insufficiency.
Data from UK CF Registry (2012) and McCormick et al. (2002).

1.5.3 Modifiers of CF phenotype

Even amongst patients with the same CF genotype there is considerable variability in disease progression. The reasons for this are multi-factorial, and include social and environmental factors, such as access to specialist healthcare and compliance with treatment regimens (Figure 1.9). Modifier genes have been postulated to play an important role in this individual disease variability. Modifier genes are polymorphisms that provide genetic variation in all individuals (i.e. what kind of cytokine response we have to a standard stimulus, etc.), but which in CF may have important implications for the response to infection and inflammation.

A number of modifier genes have been reported that may affect the severity of the clinical phenotype in a variety of ways. These include proteins that CFTR interacts with directly, such as other ion channels in the epithelial membrane, as well genes that act indirectly on the CF phenotype, such as those related to antigen processing and host defence. A list of possible modifier genes is given in Table 1.2. Most of these remain putative, and evidence from different populations is often contradictory. Of the proposed genes, the most convincing evidence for modifier effects exists for TGF-β (a cytokine involved in cell proliferation and differentiation and the regulation of fibrosis) and mannose-linding lectin (MBL) 2 (a component of the innate immune system that binds micro-organisms and promotes phagocytosis).

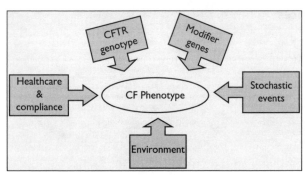

Figure 1.9 Potential determinants of CF phenotype.

Table 1.2 Proposed CF modifier genes

Category	Effect	Examples
Ion and water transport	Ion channels	• ENaC • Alternative Cl⁻ and K⁺ channels
	Ion channel activation	• β_2-AR
Immunity and airway defence	Antigen presentation	• HLA locus
	Innate defences	• Mannose-binding lectin 2 • Nitric oxide synthases
	Inflammation cascade (cytokines)	• TNFα • IL-8 • IL-10
	Neutrophil regulation	• IFRD1
	Mucins	• MUC5AC
Lung injury and repair	Proteases and anti-proteases	• Neutrophil elastase • α_1-antitrypsin • α_1-antichymotrypsin
	Oxidants/anti-oxidants	• Glutathione S-transferase (also linked to liver disease)
	Tissue growth factors	• TGF-β
	Toxic cell injury Smooth muscle tone	• Acid sphingomyelinase • Endothelin Receptor A (EDNRA)
Intra-cellular processing of CFTR		• Heat shock proteins (hsp70)

References

Boucher RC. Airway surface dehydration in cystic fibrosis: pathogenesis and therapy. *Ann Rev Med* 2007;58:157–70.

Collaco JM. Update on gene modifiers in cystic fibrosis. *Curr Opin Pulm Med*. 2008;14:559–66.

Doring G. Cystic fibrosis and innate immunity: how chloride channels provoke lung disease. *Cellular Microbiology* 2009;11:208–16.

Guggino WB. New insights into cystic fibrosis: molecular switches that regulate CFTR. *Nat Rev Mol Cell Biol* 2006;74:26–36.

McCormick J. Demographics of the UK cystic fibrosis population: implications for screening. *Eur J Hum Genet* 2002;10:583–90.

Rowe S.M. Cystic fibrosis. *N Engl J Med* 2005;352:1992–2001.

UK Cystic Fibrosis Registry. Annual data report 2012. http://www.cftrust.org.uk

Chapter 2

Diagnosis and process of care

Steve Cunningham

Key points

- Newborn screening programmes generally test for raised immune reactive trypsin (IRT) on blood taken within the first week of life, with a subsequent test for CF gene mutations if IRT is elevated
- Clinical diagnosis is most common in those with recurrent respiratory infection and poor weight gain in the first year of life
- CF may also present later in life with more subtle, but troublesome, respiratory infection, recurrent pancreatitis, or infertility
- CF is a clinical diagnosis, supported by an abnormal sweat chloride level on sweat testing
- Genetic analysis may help confirm a diagnosis of CF, but the very large number of mutations now identified make some genotype/phenotype relationships difficult to predict
- Patients with CF require regular review by health professionals trained in CF care
- Patients with CF may inadvertently share respiratory organisms and consideration should be given as to how to minimize this risk during hospital contact.
- Annual review is an important event in the care of patients with CF, enabling a multidisciplinary perspective on the rate of disease progression and plans made to slow this decline
- Transition to adult services should begin in early teens, actively involve patients and parents, and provide plenty of opportunity for transfer of information across teams

2.1 Clinical presentation

For details of newborn screening, see section 2.3.

Cystic fibrosis (CF) classically presents with failure to thrive and recurrent respiratory infection in the first few months of life. Clinical features at diagnosis and timing of presentation depend to a significant extent on patient genotype. The understanding of genotype/phenotype relationships is still evolving, but broadly divide into those with pancreatic sufficiency (c 15%) and insufficiency (c 85%).

2.1.1 Newborn

Meconium Ileus is an obstruction of the terminal ileum with inspissated meconium (see Chapter 7). It occurs in the first few days of life, and usually requires surgery to remove both the obstruction and any associated necrotic intestine.

Meconium ileus is a presenting feature in around 20% of infants with CF. 80% of cases of meconium ileus occur in patients subsequently diagnosed with CF.

Meconium ileus does not occur more frequently in any particular CF genotype.

2.1.2 **Young children**

Patients presenting in the first 5 years of life tend to be pancreatic insufficient. Malabsorption makes adequate weight gain difficult (unless weight is maintained by a voracious appetite and frequent stooling). Failure to thrive in such individuals is usually associated with recurrent respiratory infection. In many countries, with the advent of newborn screening (discussed later) such a presentation is now uncommon and often more subtle presentations take place. In areas without newborn screening a high level of suspicion should prompt sweat testing in any infant with poor growth and/or recurrent respiratory symptoms.

2.1.3 **Older children and young adults**

Presentation in older children and young adults tends to occur in those with pancreatic sufficiency, so-called 'milder' genotypes, or in those where classical symptoms and signs have not been appreciated by parents or clinical staff. Pancreatic sufficient genotypes may present with recurrent respiratory infection (sometimes unusual community acquired respiratory infections, particularly atypical mycobacteria), productive cough and bronchiectasis, chronic pancreatitis, diabetes, or infertility in males.

'Asthma' that is poorly responsive to treatment and/or associated with sputum production should raise suspicion of CF. A high index of suspicion should also be maintained for presumed diagnoses (e.g. tuberculosis with bronchiectasis) that may in fact be CF.

2.1.4 **Third decade onward**

Diagnosis in the third decade and older often follows the investigation of grumbling respiratory infections (particularly with unusual organisms and associated finger clubbing), chronic pancreatitis, diabetes, gallstones, recurrent nasal polyps, or couple infertility treatment (with male infertility from congenital absence of the *vas deferens*, CBAVD). A small proportion present with liver disease (varices, splenomegaly) without obvious signs in the chest.

Some patients have been diagnosed following the diagnosis of their child (or a relative's) identified by newborn screening.

2.2 **Diagnosis**

2.2.1 **CF is a clinical diagnosis**

Recurrent respiratory infection, with the associated development of bronchiectasis and progressive decline in respiratory function, associated with malabsorption, diabetes, liver disease, pancreatitis, nasal polyps, sinusitis, and male infertility, is consistent with the diagnosis. A positive sweat test and/or two functional mutations of the CF gene confirm the diagnosis. The sweat test is abnormal in nearly all cases, although results may fall within a normal/borderline range in pancreatic sufficient genotypes throughout life, but particularly in the first year of life.

2.2.2 **CFTR genetic variants**

The CF gene has multiple (>1900) possible mutations, some of which are not associated with clinical CF disease. The function of the gene mutation (see Chapter 1) may be sufficient for infants to be highlighted by newborn screening programs (with raised immunoreactive trypsin and rare gene mutations identified on extended gene testing), but without known clinical consequences. The future health of such infants is unknown, and they should not be regarded as having CF (as it is a clinical, not genetic diagnosis), but should be medically monitored to identify any early signs of CFTR dysfunction. Such infants have been called 'pre CF' (suggesting that CF will occur one day) or 'atypical CF' but the current suggested terminology is CFSPID (CF screen positive, inconclusive diagnosis), given the social and financial implications of a diagnosis of CF.

2.2.3 **Sweat test**

The sweat test remains the gold standard for confirmation of the clinical diagnosis (see Box 2.1). The salt content of sweat in CF is higher than non-CF individuals, because of the failure of chloride and sodium reabsorption in sweat ducts with deficient CFTR. Parents of young infants with CF not infrequently have noted that their child 'tastes' salty when kissing them. The sweat test is a test to induce and collect sweat, in which sodium, chloride, and/or conductance can be measured (see Figure 2.1). Infants generally are 6 weeks of age before they can reliably produce satisfactory sweat volumes to be tested, although testing may be possible once an infant is 48 hours old.

2.2.4 **Interpretation of sweat test**

Sweat chloride is more reliable than sweat sodium for diagnostic purposes and is considered a better discriminator for use in a reference range (see Table 2.1). An abnormal result should always be confirmed with a second test. A normal result in someone with a strong clinical suspicion of CF should also be repeated. Sweat chloride levels increase with age: lower levels may be considered suspicious in infancy.

2.2.5 **Interference with sweat test**

Contamination is a common cause of interference with the test. Measurement of sweat electrolytes by inexperienced staff leads to more frequent sampling errors, both positive and negative.

Box 2.1 Sweat test methods

Macroduct system
- Pilocarpine (a parasympathetic stimulant) induces sweat production by iontophoresis on arm or back
- Collects sweat into a small coil (minimum >15μL in 30 minutes)
- Macroduct preferred over Gibson and Cooke
- Needs experienced technician (>10 per year) and quality control

Gibson and Cooke (1959)
- Replaced previous method of placing the patient in plastic bags filled with hotwater bottles
- Pilocarpine iontophoresis as with macroduct
- Sweat is collected on a pad (gauze or filter paper)
- If sufficient weight of sweat is collected (>75mg in 30 minutes), sweat sodium and chloride will be measured

Conductance
- Measurement of sweat conductivity
- May be used for screening
- Not recommended for diagnostic purposes, and positive tests (Cl⁻ >50 mmol/l) should be referred for macroduct testing

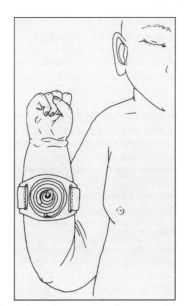

Figure 2.1 Sweat testing. Ionto-electrophoresis sweat collection into duct collecting system. Illustration by Bethany Maslen.

Table 2.1 Sweat chloride levels
<40 mmol/l Generally not considered consistent with a diagnosis of CF (though it does happen in some rare cases)
40–60 mmol/l Considered 'borderline', i.e. requires further evaluation and may be associated with pancreatic sufficient disease or may develop into clinical CF over time
>60 mmol/l Consistent with a diagnosis of CF

Conditions that affect body sodium or water concentration (i.e. malnutrition, nephrogenic diabetes insipidus) or control (i.e. mineralocorticoids) may be associated with anomalous sweat test results.

2.3 **Screening for CF**

Screening methodologies have predominantly focused on identifying individuals with severe functional loss of CFTR likely to have clinical CF in early life, although some screening methodologies inadvertently identify individuals with milder degrees of function, where the clinical course is less clear.

2.3.1 **Newborn screening**

Newborn screening for CF began to develop in earnest in the early 1980s with the recognition that residual exocrine pancreatic function could be assessed by the measurement of immunoreactive trypsin (IRT) on a blood spot from the newborn infant. The IRT continues to be used in most newborn screening programmes for CF as a screening test before the same sample is subsequently assessed for CF gene mutations.

There are many variations to newborn screening schedules adapting to methodological dilemmas (see Box 2.2), but typically a blood spot from a newborn infant (usually taken on day 2–6) will be tested for IRT. Infants with an IRT above a declared population cut-off (often ≥99.0% of population IRT), will subsequently have the blood spot screened for a range of CF gene mutations (from 1–31) specific to the mutations most prevalent in the local population. If two CF mutations are identified a diagnosis of CF is made and the family contacted.

If only one CF gene mutation is identified at initial screening some screening programs may subsequently recall infants for a further IRT measurement at 1 month. If the second IRT is high (usually ≥99.9% of population IRT), infants are referred for sweat testing and possible further genetic testing: such infants may be identified not to have CF (false positives), to have a CF gene outside the initial genetic test panel (particularly from minority ethnic groups), or a rare genotype with an unclear prognosis ('CFTR gene variants').

Newborn screening outcomes

Approximately 20% of infants with CF will be identified following a diagnosis of meconium ileus at birth. Newborn screening programmes may identify up to 80% of the remaining CF population. The health benefits of newborn screening programmes for CF have been less readily demonstrated than many would have hoped. There are improvements in the nutritional status of infants, which continue through childhood to 5 years of age, but are less distinct thereafter. More ambiguous is the benefit to pulmonary status which remains unproven. The psychological benefit to parents of an early diagnosis must be balanced by the intrusion of a life-limiting diagnosis during early bonding.

Box 2.2 Newborn screening methodology dilemmas

The number of infants identified by screening and the number of false positive and false negatives will be determined by variations in:

Where to place the population IRT cut-off percentage
• A higher percentage improves specificity but reduces sensitivity of test

What to do with heterozygous single CF genetic results
• The sensitivity of the genetic panel to identify infants with disease in the local population will depend on the size of the panel and the multicultural make-up of the local population

Whether to recall for repeat IRT
• Recalling reduces false positives (from sweat testing all raised IRT/single mutation at first round), but has significant number of false negatives with associated parental anxiety

What to do with two raised IRT
• Sweat testing may fail to identify an infant with a mild CF mutation. As a result it is not possible to confirm definitively to parents that their infant will not develop CF
• Extended genetic testing may identify additional mutations in CFTR, although the phenotype of rare mutations are often poorly described

Clinicians should make themselves aware of the date of introduction of newborn screening in their area, and the likely increased probability of CF diagnosis in those with recurrent respiratory symptoms who were born before screening was introduced.

2.3.2 Pregnancy-associated screening

Antenatal screening for CF can be population-based on a pre-conceptual or antenatal basis, or offered to a targeted population with a family history of CF.

Pre-conception screening

This has not been largely adopted because uptake is generally poor. Many couples either have not heard of CF or consider it relatively uncommon or of limited relevance to them pre-conceptually. Uptake is generally <40% and is not considered cost-effective.

Antenatal screening

Antenatal screening is considered to fulfil classic WHO criteria for use of a population screening test. The only routine regional use of antenatal screening was in Edinburgh, UK from 1991–2003, and was associated with a 65% reduction in diagnosis of CF in the local population. The programme ceased with the introduction of newborn screening.

Pregnancy screening in those with a family history

Couples who have a family history of CF may wish to identify the risk of having a child with CF by pre-conceptual screening of both partners. Where a CF mutation is identified in both partners, there will be a 1 in 4 risk of a pregnancy being affected by CF (see Figure 1.1). Couples with a 1 in 4 risk may opt to continue with the accepted risk, to undergo genetic screening of embryos by pre-implantation diagnosis, or to have chorionic villous genetic screening of the foetus at 11–12 weeks' gestation with a view to termination of an affected fetus (see Chapter 12).

2.4 Practical organization of care

In the UK, care is organized to be consistent with the Cystic Fibrosis Trust Standards of Care.

2.4.1 Outpatient

Regular review of patients with CF by professionals with an expert knowledge of the disease improves health outcomes. Outpatient review is typically once per month for young children or those with advanced disease, reducing to a minimum of 3 monthly in those who are generally well.

Health professionals who should contribute to the regular review are:

- Doctor with an expert knowledge of CF
- Nurse specialist for CF
- Pharmacist
- Psychologist
- Respiratory physiologist
- Respiratory physiotherapist
- Specialist dietitian
- Social worker

Nosocomial cross-infection of patients with CF may occur during hospital contact. In some reports, multi-resistant strains of typical CF respiratory organisms have become endemic across clinic populations, prompting a reappraisal of clinic models in recent years (see Box 2.3).

2.4.2 **Routine clinic review**

Signs and symptoms in CF are often subtle early in the disease progression. Recognition of change requires regular close monitoring by those experienced in CF care. See Box 2.4 for a summary of important aspects to be addressed at clinic review.

Clinic microbiology review

Oral antibiotics

- Most commonly given at high dose for prolonged courses (typically 14 days) appropriate to the most recent and/or most frequently identified organism on sputum/cough swab culture

Intravenous antibiotics

- Reserved for infection responding poorly to oral antibiotics or in those with regular sputum production/bronchiectasis or where there is a rapid loss of respiratory function (see Chapter 5)

Long-term antibiotics

- Consider if persistent growth of organisms on cough swab or sputum (see Chapter 4)

2.4.3 **Inpatient**

Most admissions to hospital are for intravenous antibiotic therapy to treat a chest infection (see Chapter 5). The same cross-infection concerns during outpatient contact apply also to inpatient care.

Box 2.3 Types of clinic model

Cepacia-only segregation
Segregate only patients colonised with B. cepacia—hold separate clinic days for B. cepacia patients. All other patients attend together on another day.

Microbiological cohorting
Segregate clinics into cohorts of B. cepacia, multi-resistant Pseudomonas aeruginosa (Pa), other Pa, non-Pa—i.e. 4 clinic days.

Individual segregation
Segregation of all patients from each other during clinic visits; this accepts that knowledge of lower airway organisms is poor in many patients with CF who do not expectorate, and the safest approach is to assume that all patients may have organisms potentially cross-infectious to others.

In this clinic model, patients are allocated an individual time for attendance, are provided with a clinic room which they remain in for their whole appointment and through which health professionals rotate to consult the patient (as opposed to the traditional model of patients rotating through rooms to consult health professionals). Clinic room surfaces are cleaned between patients, and health professionals must adhere to scrupulous cleaning of hands and instruments.

With the better understanding of the cross infection risk of Mycobacteria abscessus and other organisms, this has become the clinic style of choice.

Box 2.4 Clinic review

Chest
Recent symptoms

- Cough/breathlessness/wheeze/sputum production/haemoptysis
- Recent antibiotics and response (or lack of)

Auscultation

- Crepitations are typically a feature of advanced, and often irreversible, CF lung disease, and significant respiratory infection often occurs in the absence of chest signs in patients with CF
- Wheeze may occur in those with concurrent asthma, secretions in the airways or allergic bronchopulmonary aspergillosis (ABPA)

Pulmonary function

- Usually spirometry at clinic visits. Loss of function should be as slow as possible. 10% reduction between visits considered important to regain, usually with intravenous antibiotics unless rapidly gained by oral antibiotics. Deteriorating rate of decline in pulmonary function may be smoothed by use of mucolytics (i.e. dornase alfa) in addition to regular chest physiotherapy and antibiotics

Physiotherapy

- Adherence and technique should be checked and alternate techniques suggested if required
- Microbiological culture of cough swab / sputum

Abdomen and nutrition
Weight and height (often as BMI)

- Plotted and reviewed for rate of change in children, and weight gain/loss in adults

Recent symptoms

- Abdominal pain/discomfort
- Stool frequency and colour

Palpation

- Fecal masses are most frequently palpated in the right lower quadrant—patients with chronic masses can often point them out to you

Nutritional supplements

- Oral (often poorly tolerated/adhered to)
- Overnight or daytime bolus feeds may be given by nasogastric tube or via gastrostomy

Diabetes
- Typically subtle signs (see Chapter 8). Diabetes may only be present during a respiratory exacerbation
- Suspect where there are increased respiratory infections and/or weight loss/poorer gain than expected, particularly in those over 10 years of age

(continued)

Box 2.4 Continued

Liver disease
- Often not associated with symptoms and detected by abnormal liver function tests at annual review. Usually first palpated as a large liver. May be associated with varices and haematemesis, or portal hypertension with large spleen and abdominal discomfort

Polyps/sinusitis
- Recurrent headache or frontal pressure
- Nasal obstruction
- Loss of sense of smell and taste

Bone and joint disease
- Joint pain/reduced mobility
- Recent bone fracture
- Poor bone mineralization may occur in patients with CF with poor mobility (compounded by vitamin K malabsorption). DXA scans and supplementation of vitamin K and Adcal may help

- Patients should be segregated and have no, or minimal, contact, and should not share the same area for physiotherapy without the area being cleaned and ventilated thoroughly
- Patients and carers should perform hand-washing when moving between areas

2.5 **Annual review**

The patient with CF requires careful review at least once each year as the condition is both multidisciplinary and multisystem. Disease progression is often subtle and slow. Careful attention to detail may identify and impede acceleration in speed of decline.

The annual review enables members of the multidisciplinary team to reflect on the rate of change for systems individually and collectively, and consider how their discipline can modify outcomes in the subsequent year. This usually requires a systematic review of each of the systems affected by CF (see Table 2.2). Annual review is also a good opportunity to ensure that up-to-date screening has taken place for development of important complications (e.g. diabetes, osteoporosis).

2.5.1 **Annual review outcomes**

The annual review discussion should bring together the perspective of all disciplines and may include consideration of (but not limited to) the following:

- Have unusual organisms been looked for?
- Should there be discussions about change in strategy for next year (e.g., regular IV antibiotic treatment/trial of NG tube feeding, etc.)?
- Is rate of deterioration of pulmonary function greater than expected and does this warrant further investigation (CT chest, bronchoscopy, etc.)?
- Has consideration been given to age-related issues, such as discussion for males on infertility and for females on need for contraception?

Table 2.2 CF annual review—typical investigations

Assessments depend on age and status of the patient, but typically include most or all of the following:

Blood samples

- Full blood count
- Urea and electrolytes, calcium, magnesium, and phosphate
- Random blood glucose and glucose-tolerance test
- Liver function tests
- Total IgE, specific IgE to aspergillus and aspergillus precipitins
- Other immunoglobulins: IgG, IgA, IgM
- Pseudomonas antibodies
- Vitamins A, D, E, and K

Pulmonary function

- Spirometry and reversibility to bronchodilator
- Lung volumes
- Transfer factor
- SpO_2 on air

Exercise tolerance

- Measure of exercise tolerance (i.e. 6-minute walk, 3-minute step test, or cardiopulmonary exercise testing)

Respiratory review

- Change in symptom frequency over past year (cough, respiratory exacerbation, perception of breathlessness)
- Number, frequency, and type of antibiotic courses
- Sputum frequency, volume, and colour
- Evidence of haemoptysis

Microbiology review

- Type of organism, frequency of occurrence, change in sensitivity patterns
- Culture for detection of unusual pathogens (aspergillus and mycobacteria)

GI/nutrition review

- Height and weight centiles/z scores with BMI
- Review of dietary intake with food diary
- Review of dose and frequency of pancreatic enzyme supplements
- Liver ultrasound (annually if abnormal liver function tests or as clinically indicated)
- Bone densitometry every 3 years from early teens

Pharmacy review

- Review of current medication, and possible interactions
- Review adherence, and discuss barriers and solutions
- Education about the role of different medications
- Discuss patient preferences, and alternatives (where appropriate)

(continued)

Table 2.2 Continued
Psychology and social review

- Review of psychological adaptation to disease and changes in condition during past year
- Is patient/family enabled to access sufficient benefits they are entitled to receive?
- Are schools/work places provided with sufficient information to sustain their continued support during periods of health-related absence?
- Appropriate information on sexual health and reproduction
- Life expectancy and outcomes

2.6 **CFTR variant clinics**

Newborn screening programmes have identified a significant proportion of infants who do not have a classical diagnosis of CF, but for whom there is a high index of suspicion that they may develop CF in the future. In Edinburgh, we have developed a paediatric CFTR variant clinic that reviews infants and children identified by newborn screening. Such individuals would typically have either a raised IRT, one gene defect, and a borderline sweat test, or two gene defects of unknown/limited phenotypic description and a low or borderline sweat test. Such children are not labelled as CF, but are reviewed on a regular basis (minimum annual) by a CF doctor. A sweat test is repeated at age 5 years or sooner as clinically indicated. With a clinical diagnosis of CF children move across to a routine CF clinic and multidisciplinary team.

2.7 **Transition**

Children with CF grow up with a close cohort of multidisciplinary professionals providing care on a regular basis, where these professionals are a constant and (hopefully) friendly aspect of life for the nascent young adults as they approach the age of transition to adult services.

Transition to adult services is most often a significant wrench for parents, who have invested many years of faith in one group of professionals who have to relinquish (often reluctantly) not only the close relationship with professionals, but also some degree of parental responsibility for ongoing care. See also Chapter 10 for a discussion of the psychological challenges of transition.

Young adults transition to adult services in a period between the 15th and 18th birthdays, most typically when 16–17 years of age.

2.7.1 **The transition process**

Age 12 years (depending on individual maturity)

Young adults should be encouraged to become more actively involved in providing details of symptoms and treatments.

Age 14 years onwards

Some young adults may benefit from seeing professionals on their own, with their parents joining consultations for a summary at the end. Young adults can begin to be invited to participate more actively in healthcare decisions, and in balancing the risk and benefits of choices.

Box 2.5 Transition process

Visit 1 An initial transition clinic takes place with the paediatric team alone, where the process of transition is discussed, and young adults are invited to express their expectations and concerns.

Visit 2 Immediately preceding the second transition clinic, the two multidisciplinary teams have a meeting to discuss the individual patients who are to transfer care that year, using a full written summary provided by the paediatrician. Pairs of professionals from each sub-discipline then go to meet the young adults with CF (and their parents) to review previous progress and to discuss a plan for future care (it is particularly important that transition is not associated with a step change in policy).

Visit 3 In the third clinic meeting a similar process occurs, but this time hosted by the adult care team at the adult unit, with the adult teams taking the lead during consultations.

Visit 4 In the fourth and final clinic young adults meet with the adult team at the adult unit, without a paediatric presence, and the transition is considered complete.

Age 15–18 years

A formal process of transition takes place to transfer care to adult services. There are many models. In the UK, it is recommended that a process of transfer takes place over the course of 4 clinic appointments in a period of covering 6 months (Box 2.5).

At the completion of visit 4 no further advice or inpatient care is directed by the paediatric team, and the process of transition is considered complete.

References

Castellani C, et al. European best practice guidelines for CF neonatal screening. *J Cyst Fibrosis* 2009;8:153–7.

Farrell PM, et al. Guidelines for diagnosis of CF in newborns through older adults: CF Foundation consensus report. *J Pediatrics* 2008;153:S4–S14.

Gibson LE, Cooke RE. A test for concentration of electrolytes in sweat in CF of the pancreas utilizing pilocarpine iontophoresis. *Pediatrics* 1959;23:545–9.

Standards for the Clinical Care of Children and Adults with Cystic Fibrosis in the UK, 2nd edn. UK CF Trust, 2011.

Transition Medicine Clinical Standards. CF. Royal College of Physicians of Edinburgh, 2008. <http://www.rcpe.ac.uk

Chapter 3

Microbiology of CF lung disease

John Govan and Andrew Jones

Key points

- Bacterial lung infections are the predominant cause of restricted quality of life and life expectancy of CF patients
- If infection is allowed to become chronic, eradication of bacterial pathogens is virtually impossible
- Major CF pathogens show striking adaptation in genotype and phenotype to the lung environment
- CF lung infection involves a mixed bacterial population of facultative aerobes and obligate anaerobes
- Mucoid, alginate-producing *Pseudomonas aeruginosa* are the most prevalent and important CF pathogens. The mucoid phenotype is associated with bacterial mutations and formation of biofilms, and is characteristic of chronic infection
- Early aggressive antipseudomonal therapy at the onset of infection offers the best chance of eradication or delay in the onset of chronic infection
- Many CF pathogens are either innately resistant to multiple antibiotics or are able to acquire resistance. Effective antibiotic therapy is also hampered by slow bacterial growth within biofilms and, with the exception of nebulized/inhaled antibiotics, by poor antibiotic penetration into CF airways

27

3.1 Introduction

In individuals with CF, respiratory infections start early in life and are the major cause of morbidity and mortality. Historically, chronic pulmonary infections were considered to be caused by a surprisingly limited range of micro-organisms. Recently non-culture methodologies have indicated that the microbiome is more complex than previously believed, comprising a multiple interacting microbial community.

Unlike the healthy lung, respiratory infections in CF tend to be persistent, often involving phenotypic change in the organisms themselves. This is strikingly demonstrated in the emergence of the mucoid colonial phenotype in *P. aeruginosa*. Organisms may colonize the lungs asymptomatically; at other times, the same organism may be responsible for acute pulmonary exacerbations and uncontrolled inflammation leading to progressive lung damage. Treatments are aimed at:

1. Preventing acquisition of infection
2. Early eradication of new organisms
3. Resolution of acute exacerbations

4. Maintaining or preventing loss of lung function by regular antibiotic administration. Eradication of chronic infection, in particular that caused by mucoid *P. aeruginosa,* is notoriously difficult, if not impossible

The sequence of infecting pulmonary organisms follows a classical chronological course, illustrated in Figure 3.1. In early childhood, *S. aureus* is the organism most frequently isolated, with a prevalence of approximately 50% by the age of 10 years. Non-capsulate *Haemophilus influenzae* is also isolated frequently during childhood, but less so in older children and adults, in whom the major pathogen is *P. aeruginosa.* Other significant pathogens, albeit with a relatively lower prevalence, include *Burkholderia cepacia* complex bacteria (BCC) and non-tuberculous mycobacteria (NTM). Innately multi-resistant opportunistic pathogens such as *Stenotrophomonas maltophilia* and *Achromobacter xylosoxidans* are also encountered. In addition, many species of obligate anaerobic bacteria have recently been identified in the airways of CF patients (see Table 3.1).

3.1.1 **Microbiological methods**

The role of the microbiology laboratory is crucial to ensure optimum care for those with CF including assisting therapeutic decision making and infection control practices. Culture of CF pathogens and accurate identification can be challenging and is aided by experience of CF microbiology, the use of selective culture media for specific pathogens, and the availability of national guidelines on laboratory standards for processing microbiological samples. Long-term reliance on bacterial culture as a primary tool in diagnosis is also being challenged by the development of culture-independent techniques based on detecting bacterial RNA or DNA. Not only do such techniques provide more rapid diagnoses but their ability to recognize the presence of potential pathogens with demanding growth requirements suggests that the CF lung contains a complex and diverse microbiome of bacteria whose precise composition may differ between patients. Severe lung disease, for example, is associated with reduction in the diversity of the lung microbiome. These unexpected findings provide many challenges to the CF microbiologist including the unanswered questions of what drives bacterial diversity in individual patients, how potential pathogens interact, and importantly, whether we are directing antibiotic therapy at the right pathogens.

3.2 *Staphylococcus aureus*

3.2.1 **Epidemiology**

S. aureus is frequently found in the respiratory tract secretions of CF patients, either as a sole pathogen or in combination with other bacteria (Figure 3.1). Chronic *S. aureus* infection is particularly common in children. Family members may share genetically identical *S. aureus* clones with CF patients, suggesting they may represent a source of *S. aureus* acquisition: one-third of healthy non-CF adults are nasal carriers of *S. aureus*, and rates of carriage are twice as high in individuals with CF. With increasing age, *S. aureus* is eclipsed by *P. aeruginosa* as the most commonly isolated micro-organism in the CF lung. Small colony variants of *S. aureus* may be overgrown by mucoid *P. aeruginosa*, therefore the additional use of selective media for staphylococci such as mannitol salt agar or Columbia/colistimethate sodium nalidixic acid media is recommended for the culture of CF respiratory tract secretions.

3.2.2 **Virulence factors**

S. aureus isolates from CF patients may express several virulence factors: membrane-damaging toxins such as leukotoxins, hemolysins, or the Panton–Valentine leukocidin (PVL). PVL is a cytolytic toxin that forms pores in the membranes of leukocytes, leading to cell death. PVL

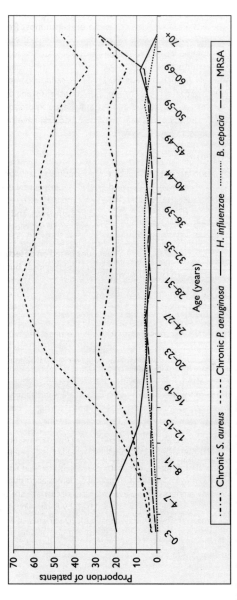

Figure 3.1 Age-dependent prevalence of bacteria in the CF lung. (UK CF Registry 2012).

Table 3.1 Major microbial species in the CF airways
Facultative aerobic bacteria
• *Staphylococcus aureus* and MRSA • *Haemophilus influenzae* • *Pseudomonas aeruginosa* • *Burkholderia cepacia* complex bacteria • Non-tuberculous mycobacteria • Other gram-negative bacteria: e.g. *Stenotrophomonas maltophila*, *Achromobacter (Alcaligenes) xylosoxidans*, and *Ralstonia*, *Pandoraea*, *Inquilinus*, and *Cupriavidus* species
Obligate anaerobic bacteria
• e.g. *Prevotella*, *Peptosteptococcus*, *Actinomyces*, *Veilonella*, *Streptococcus*, *Bacteroides*, *Gemella*, *Propionibacterium*, and *Wolinella* spp.
Fungi
• *Aspergillus fumigatus*

is more commonly encountered in, although not exclusive to, MRSA (meticillin-resistant *S. aureus*) strains. Surface factors and extracellular proteins (protein A, capsules) may inhibit phagocytosis, and enzymes such as superoxide dismutase may inactivate neutrophil-derived oxygen radicals and thereby impair innate antimicrobial defences. Small colony variants, so called because of their appearance on agar plates, are associated with greater persistence in the airways and greater adherence to respiratory epithelium.

3.2.3 **Clinical consequence**

S. aureus commonly colonizes the lung early in life and causes recurrent infection in some CF individuals.

3.2.4 **Treatment**

There are two possible approaches to *S. aureus* infection in CF. The first is to provide prophylactic flucloxacillin to newborns with CF to reduce the prevalence of *S. aureus* infection and associated inflammation, at least for the first 3 years of life. Evidence for this approach is limited, and there are concerns that continuous antibiotics may predispose to a higher rate of *P. aeruginosa* acquisition. The second approach is to conduct regular monitoring of airway secretions microbiologically and provide prompt treatment of symptomatic *S. aureus*. The benefits of one approach over the other have not been clearly defined and are often a matter of local preference. Treatment of acute exacerbations involving *S. aureus* is described in Chapter 5.

3.3 **MRSA**

Strains of *S. aureus* that possess the mecA gene exhibit resistance to meticillin, flucloxacillin, and frequently other common anti-staphylococal antibiotics; however, they are usually susceptible to vancomycin. The prevalence of MRSA infection in CF has increased over the past decade, particularly in North America, in line with increases in MRSA colonization both in hospitals and in the community.

3.3.1 **Clinical consequence**

MRSA infection is associated with more frequent intravenous antibiotic courses, increased hospitalization, and lower lung function values in CF children and adults.

3.3.2 **Treatment**

Many CF centres now adopt an aggressive policy towards MRSA infection, with multiple attempts at eradication. A variety of eradication regimens are used in practice and these can produce sustained eradication in over 80% of patients. Up to 3 attempts at eradication, using the same or different therapies, are recommended. An example of an eradication regimen is given in Box 3.1.

Nebulized vancomycin has also been used in eradication regimens at some CF centres. This is given 2–4 times daily for the first five days of treatment as 250 mg (or 4 mg/kg in children) diluted to 4 ml in sterile water. A dry-powder formulation of vancomycin delivered by inhalation is also undergoing evaluation.

Eradication also involves elimination of non-respiratory carriage. The following steps are recommended for 5 days:

- Nasal carriage: Topical mupirocin 2% or vancomycin cream 2% four times daily
- Skin carriage: 4% chlorhexidine bath/shower on alternate days
- Oropharyngeal carriage: vancomycin 5% lozenges qds or vancomycin 2% paste/gel four times daily

3.4 **Haemophilus influenza**

Non-typable *H. influenzae* is a common commensal in the healthy human upper respiratory tract. In the CF lung these bacteria can play a major role in pulmonary exacerbations in young children. Infection tends to be more acute/periodic and less chronic than that for other organisms. Successful laboratory culture of *H. influenzae*, particularly in the presence of other CF pathogens, is aided by homogenization and dilution of sputum, and by specific culture media such as chocolate agar (supplemented with bacitracin) incubated anaerobically. *H. influenzae* may chronically colonize the CF lung; penetration of the bacteria into

---

Box 3.1 Example MRSA eradication regimen for CF patients

1st line. 6 weeks of both of:
- Rifampicin 5–10 mg/kg (max 450 mg) (children and adults <50 kg), 600 mg (adults) PO 12 hrly
- Fusidic acid 15 mg/kg (<1yr), 250 mg (1-5 yrs), 500 mg (5–12 yrs) or 750mg (>12 yrs) PO 8 hrly

2nd line. 6 weeks of 2 of the following antibiotics depending on sensitivities: -
- Doxycycline (>12 yrs) 200 mg first dose, then 100–200 mg PO once daily
- Trimethoprim 4 mg/kg (max 200 mg) PO 12 hrly
- Rifampicin* (see above for dosing)
- Fusidic acid* (see above for dosing)

3rd line. 2 weeks of either of the following regimens, followed by 4 weeks of a 2nd line oral combination
- Teicoplanin 10 mg/kg (max 400 mg) IV 12 hrly for 3 doses then once daily
OR
- Linezolid 10 mg/kg (max 600 mg) PO 8hrly (<12 hrs) or 12 hrly (>12 yrs)—this should only be used under supervision of a microbiologist, and its use is limited to 14 consecutive days

epithelial cells may contribute to persistence of *H. influenzae* in CF. Pulmonary exacerbations due to *H. influenzae* are associated with increased inflammatory markers and with high bacterial counts in sputum. Antibiotic treatment of exacerbations due to *H. influenzae* must take account of the presence or absence of β-lactamase-producing strains (and *P. aeruginosa*) whose presence will affect susceptibility to amoxicillin.

H. influenzae is associated with fewer pulmonary exacerbations in older CF patients. It should be noted that strains that are found in the CF lung are non-capsulated. Therefore, in individuals with CF, application of the *H. influenzae* type B vaccine does not protect from *Haemophilus* acquisition.

3.5 **Pseudomonas aeruginosa**

3.5.1 **Background**

P. aeruginosa is a non-sporing, Gram-negative rod-shaped bacterium. It is usually motile by virtue of one or more polar flagella. These bacteria are capable of utilizing a wide variety of nutrients and are thus found in many natural environments, particularly soil and water. *P. aeruginosa* harbours a relatively large genome; the resulting genetic diversity and notorious adaptability contribute to its ability to cause a wide range of infections and its persistence in hostile environments. Most strains are intrinsically resistant to many antibiotics, are able to metabolize a wide range of carbon and nitrogen sources, and can grow in both aerobic and anaerobic environments. *P. aeruginosa* possess an armoury of bacterial virulence factors, regulated by complex systems such as quorum sensing, including LPS-endotoxin, pili, flagella, and secreted factors such as elastase, phospholipase, and two potent exotoxins, exotoxin A and exoenzyme S.

Non-mucoid and mucoid forms

In the environment, and in the majority of non-CF infections, *P. aeruginosa* exist as single, motile bacteria that form easily identified rough, green-pigmented colonies on laboratory culture. This is the so-called non-mucoid form of the organism. In the primary stages of CF airway colonization, bacterial chemotaxis towards airway mucin, and pili-mediated adhesion to specific receptors, facilitate early and often transient infections. Stimulation of the innate immune system and an enhanced host cytokine response leads to neutrophil chemotaxis to the site of infection. However, resolution of the infection is thwarted by an unusual bacterial adaptation involving production of an alginate-like polysaccharide and formation of bacterial biofilms. Within a biofilm, the action of antibiotics is reduced by slow bacterial growth; at the same time, the biofilm presents a physical barrier to efficient phagocytic killing (Figure 3.2). A persistent influx of 'frustrated phagocytes' not only fails to prevent chronic infection, but also results in the release of toxic neutrophil contents (including elastase) and progressive inflammatory damage and airway remodelling.

Chronic pseudomonas infection of the CF lung

Once mucoid *P. aeruginosa* appear in the CF lung, the organisms are seldom if ever eradicated. Children with CF who are chronically infected with *P. aeruginosa* have poorer pulmonary function, lower chest radiograph scores, and worse 10-year survival rates than uninfected CF children. In addition, the biofilm mode of growth associated with mucoid *P. aeruginosa* is associated with enhanced, but not protective, antibody production against numerous bacterial antigens, the formation of immune complexes, and large numbers of activated neutrophils in the airway lumen.

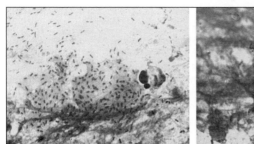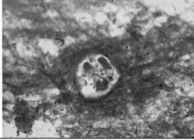

Figure 3.2 Contrasting bacterial adaptation in CF airways to frustrate a phagocyte. Gram-stains showing biofilm-mode of growth associated with resistance of mucoid alginate-producing *Pseudomonas aeruginosa* to pulmonary neutrophil (left), compared with intracellular survival of *Burkholderia cenocepacia* (right).

3.5.2 **Routes of transmission**

Since chronic *P. aeruginosa* infection plays such a dominant role in the morbidity associated with CF, every reasonable effort should be undertaken to prevent acquisition of this pathogen. However, it should also be emphasized that avoidance of all possible environmental sources of *P. aeruginosa* in the home or elsewhere is not realistic, and in addition, definitive proof that CF patients have been infected by a given contaminated environmental source is rare.

Patient segregation

During the 1990s several seminal studies provided compelling evidence of cross-infection with *P. aeruginosa* between CF patients, and demonstrated the emergence of highly transmissible 'epidemic' strains. To avoid cross-infection amongst patients, CF centres now commonly segregate CF patients with and without *P. aeruginosa* infection. In many centres patients with and without *P. aeruginosa* infection are seen in clinics held on different days of the week. Similar strategies are also recommended for the separation of other groups of CF patients infected with other pathogens, such as *B. cepacia* complex, MRSA, or NTM. The previous practice of holding summer camps and other social activities where CF patients live together for periods of time is now actively discouraged.

3.5.3 **Diagnosis**

P. aeruginosa infections are typically diagnosed using routine microbiological culture of respiratory tract secretions. The prognostic value of *P. aeruginosa* serology for antibiotic therapy in CF patients is unclear. Serological tests for *P. aeruginosa* antigens (generally ELISA assays) may be useful in non-expectorating patients, including patients younger than 6 years, in whom routine pseudomonas surveillance may yield false-negative results. Serology may also complement culture results to monitor recurrence of early *P. aeruginosa* infection. Early detection of *P. aeruginosa* colonization is beneficial, since early antibiotic treatment can be initiated before the infection becomes established. Therefore it is recommended that all CF patients, regardless of clinical status, should have a respiratory tract culture performed at least quarterly. In culture negative, symptomatic, non-expectorating young children, bronchoscopic evaluation of the lower airway may be necessary to investigate for infection with *P. aeruginosa*.

3.5.4 **Pseudomonas vaccines**

Prevention of *P. aeruginosa* infection by vaccination seems a rational strategy and might in future be achieved. However, early vaccine trials, which included individuals already colonized with *P. aeruginosa*, were stopped because of adverse immunological reactions. More recently, trials of vaccines based on exotoxin A-polysaccharide and on *Pseudomonas*-flagella have been disappointing. At present, there is no commercially available anti-pseudomonal vaccine.

3.5.5 **Early eradication therapy for *Pseudomonas***

Antibiotic therapy, initiated shortly after the confirmation of *P. aeruginosa* lung colonization, provides a promising strategy to eradicate early infection and reduce the incidence of chronic carriage. At this stage, the bacterium exhibits the non-mucoid phenotype, biofilm formation is minimal, and eradication of the pathogen is achieved in approximately 80% of patients after a single treatment. Unlike the situation in chronic *P. aeruginosa* infection (where antibiotic sensitivity tests are unhelpful), sensitivity testing of early isolates can be helpful in the choice of regimen to be used. Currently, the optimal regimen for empirical use of antibiotics has not been determined. An example of a typical treatment regimen to eradicate newly acquired *P. aeruginosa* is given in Chapter 4.

3.5.6 **Antibiotic therapy strategies**

It is virtually impossible to eradicate mucoid *P. aeruginosa* in the chronic infection state using any antibiotic therapy regimen; at best, this achieves only a reduction of *Pseudomonas* cell density within the airways. This phenomenon may have a number of explanations:

1 The reduced efficacy of nearly all antibiotics under reduced oxygen tensions. Oxygen diffusion through pseudomonas biofilms is poor, creating hypoxic zones around the bacterial colonies

2 Antibiotic binding, and hence reduced inhibitory activity, in the presence of proteins and electrolytes within CF airways

3 The consequences of a slow bacterial growth rate on the killing potential of antibiotics within biofilms

4 Sub-inhibitory concentrations of antibiotics in CF airways may negatively affect clinical outcomes by inducing pseudomonas biofilm formation and increasing the rate of mutation of hypermutable strains

Despite these challenges, reduction in bacterial cell density in the CF lung is still beneficial in reducing progressive lung damage. For example, reduction of an initial *P. aeruginosa* cell density from 10^8 to 10^6 cfu/ml represents killing of 99.0% of the bacteria. Together with the therapeutic impact of sub-inhibitory antibiotic concentrations on bacterial virulence, this seems sufficient to improve clinical outcome, reduce inflammatory parameters, increase quality of life, and improve nutritional status of the patients. High doses of antibiotics are recommended to achieve satisfactory drug concentrations at the site of infection (e.g. in sputum plugs). To obtain sufficiently high antibiotic dosages in the CF lung and improve the efficacy of antibiotic delivery, an increasing number of antibiotics (including colistimethate sodium, tobramycin, aztreonam, ciprofloxacin, and amikacin) have been or are being developed as new formulations suitable for delivery by the aerosolised route, a strategy which reduces adverse effects compared with intravenously administered antibiotics. During acute exacerbations, antibiotics should also be administered intravenously (see Chapter 5).

3.6 **Other important pathogens**

3.6.1 *Burkholderia cepacia* complex (BCC)

The early 1990s marked an important development in CF microbiology with the increasing emergence of a 'new' pathogen, known at the time as '*Pseudomonas cepacia*', and later '*Burkholderia cepacia*'. Not surprisingly, increasing concern raised by outbreaks of 'cepacia' within CF centres, and the organism's alarming potential to cause life-threatening infection, became the raison d'être for ready acceptance in the CF community of draconian measures of infection control, including strict segregation of infected patients and the need to focus research on what has turned out to be an important group of highly adaptable organisms.

Epidemiology

Following ground-breaking taxonomic studies, isolates previously described as '*B. cepacia*' now represents a group of Gram-negative bacteria comprising at least 17 distinct species, and known collectively as the *B. cepacia complex* (BCC). Individual BCC species are phenotypically identical, require specific culture media, and are identified on the basis of biochemical or DNA-based tests.

As a group, BCC are ubiquitous environmental organisms, commonly found in water and soil including the plant rhizosphere. Although the majority of the 17 BCC species have been isolated from CF individuals, ongoing epidemiological surveillance indicates that around 90% of infections in CF are caused by only two species, *Burkholderia cenocepacia* and *Burkholderia multivorans*. Although the implementation of stringent infection control measures have led to a significant reduction in prevalence (to less than 10%), the BCC remain particularly feared in the CF population.

Clinical consequence

Some strains of BCC species—in particular *B. cenocepacia*, *B. multivorans* and the closely related, but non-BCC species, *Burkholderia gladioli*—are highly transmissible. The clinical course after acquisition follows one of three patterns. It must be emphasized, however, that within individual patients the clinical course is unpredictable even in individuals infected with the same strain.

1 No deterioration in lung function or clinical condition

2 Accelerated decline in lung function (most common)

3 A rapid, fatal, and unexpected decline in lung function

This last pattern may be accompanied by fulminating pneumonia and septicaemia, and is known as the 'cepacia syndrome' (Figure 3.3). Amongst CF pathogens, cepacia syndrome represents a unique example in CF microbiology of systemic spread of a pathogen outside the lung. The syndrome is most commonly associated with *B. cenocepacia*, but is not exclusive to this species. Importantly, it is also unpredictable and may occur many years after acquisition. Host/pathogen interactions may be key to the development of cepacia syndrome. The nature of such interactions is unclear; however, accumulated evidence suggests that BCC infection primes a CF individual to react adversely to new infection with other pathogens and invasive procedures such as bronchoscopy.

Infection with *B. cenocepacia* is considered a contra-indication to lung transplantation because of the higher rates of early post-transplant mortality. BCC infection also remains a common contra-indication for inclusion in clinical trials.

In some patients, with the exception of *B. cenocepacia*, there appears to be spontaneous clearance after initial isolation of the organism, but this should not be assumed until at least

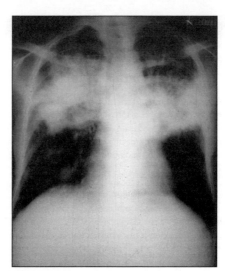

Figure 3.3 Chest X-ray of a CF patient with cepacia syndrome.

3 sequential good quality sputum cultures have been clear of the organism over a period of at least 6–12 months. Whilst there is little evidence for the beneficial effect of treatment to aid eradication, many centres offer this after initial isolation of BCC.

The mucoid/biofilm paradox

Although some BCC are capable of exopolysaccharide-mediated biofilm growth in vitro, there is little evidence that BCC species resemble mucoid *P. aeruginosa* and benefit from exopolysaccharide-enhanced biofilm growth in the CF lung. In contrast, it is likely that BCC rely on a different adaptation resembling that of the closely related, highly virulent pathogen *Burkholderia pseudomallei*, the causative agent of melioidosis. This involves intracellular survival within phagocytic cells of the immune system mediated by characteristic innate resistance of the *Burkholderia* species to cationic peptides and oxidative killing (Figure 3.2). Although most BCC species can express the mucoid phenotype, particularly when grown in the presence of mannitol and other sugar alcohols, most strains of the highly virulent species, *B. cenocepacia*, contain a mutation inhibiting exopolysaccharide synthesis. In contrast to the emergence, and apparent selection, of mucoid *P. aeruginosa* in the CF lung, the mucoid colonial phenotype of BCC is lost during chronic infection.

Treatment

Antibiotic treatment of BCC infections is difficult since the pathogen is generally resistant to many classes of antibiotics including aminoglycosides, quinolones, β-lactams, and antimicrobial peptides. Some BCC produce a highly inducible β-lactamase and are capable of using penicillin as a sole carbon source. Combinations of antibiotics, according to the minimal inhibition concentrations, are recommended. Combinations of at least 3 IV antibiotics are recommended. Those containing meropenem are most likely to be successful, usually together with one or more of tobramycin, co-trimoxazole, chloramphenicol, tetracyclines, or piperacillin-tazobactam (see Chapter 5).

3.7 **Mycobacterial infection**

3.7.1 **Epidemiology**

Non-tuberculous mycobacteria (NTM) have been detected in an increasing number of respiratory specimens from CF patients. In 2003, a prospective, cross-sectional study found a prevalence of NTM in 13% of patients at 21 US CF centres; *Mycobacterium avium* complex (72%) and *M. abscessus* (16%) were the most common NTM species. In an Israeli study, the prevalence of NTM approached 23% in CF patients, with *M. simiae* (41%), *M. abscessus* (31%), and *M. avium* complex (14%) being detected most frequently. The reasons for increased NTM infections, and in particular *M. abscessus,* in adult patients with CF are unclear. Until recently, there has been little evidence for patient-to-patient transmission. However, retrospective use of whole genome sequencing has suggested transmission of *M. abscessus* between a small number of patients attending a large UK CF centre.

3.7.2 **Clinical consequence**

Although no significant short-term effect on lung function has been demonstrated in patients with multiple positive NTM cultures, an abnormal high-resolution computed tomography (HRCT) can be suggestive of progressive lung disease. *M. abscessus* infection is a significant additional risk factor, which may be a relative contra-indication, for lung transplantation.

Specific treatment, tailored to microbiological sensitivities, should be considered in patients with NTM infection, particularly those repeatedly smear- or culture-positive, or with deteriorating clinical status or progression of changes on HRCT. The decision to treat is not trivial, since eradication regimens typically involve 3–4 oral +/- 1 nebulized antibiotic, often with significant potential toxicities, and are continued for 18–24 months. The clinical significance of NTM in CF needs to be further studied, as do the long-term effects of treatment.

3.8 *Stenotrophomonas maltophilia*

3.8.1 **Epidemiology**

S. maltophilia is another ubiquitous Gram-negative organism, found in aquatic environments, soil, and vegetation. It may be found in plumbing, including shower-heads, taps, and sinks, and is widespread in the home and in hospital. Prevalence in CF has been increasing over the last 20 years, and is between 10–20%. It is more likely to affect those with poorer clinical condition, but can also be found in patients with good lung function. Microbiological surveillance in CF homes, including the use of bacterial 'fingerprinting' has provided little evidence that a patient's home environment is associated with acquisition of *S. maltophilia.*

3.8.2 **Clinical consequence**

S. maltophilia produce few obvious virulence factors and the clinical significance of the infection is controversial. A large retrospective US study found no independent association between survival of *S. maltophilia*-infected patients compared to all others, when stratified for lung function. In individual CF patients, however, *S. maltophilia* infection may be clinically significant.

3.8.3 **Treatment**

The optimal treatment of *S. maltophilia* remains to be established; often no treatment is required if the organism is considered to be a colonizer. Despite an increasing number of resistant strains, co-trimoxazole remains the drug of choice. Minocycline shows good *in vitro* activity against *S. maltophilia,* but clinical experience is limited and it is contra-indicated in children under 12 years old. There is also good sensitivity (80%) to doxycycline. *S. maltophilia* is inherently resistant to carbapenems (imipenem, meropenem), and most strains are also resistant to aztreonam, tobramycin, piperacillin-tazobactam, and colistimethate sodium.

3.9 *Achromobacter* species

Achromobacter spp. have also been recovered from respiratory tract cultures of CF patients with increasing frequency over the last decade, the most common being *A. xylosoxidans* (previously *Alcaligenes xylosoxidans*) and *A. ruhlandii*. Transmissibility of *Achromobacter* spp. between CF patients has not yet been demonstrated. Laboratory culture and identification of *Achromobacter* presents few difficulties, but use of MacConkey agar is recommended. Accurate laboratory identification of this potential pathogen is important as it may be mistaken as a multi-resistant *P. aeruginosa*. The pathogenicity of *Achromobacter* spp. for CF patients remains largely unclear, although an association with pulmonary exacerbations has been reported. The prevalence rate for *Achromobacter* spp. varies widely between centres, but may approach between 5–10% in CF adults.

Therapy of *Achromobacter* spp. poses major problems because of intrinsic multi-resistance or fast development of new resistance. Combination therapy with 2 or 3 antibiotics according to the results of *in vitro* susceptibility testing is recommended.

3.10 **Obligate anaerobes**

Microaerobic/anaerobic conditions exist in CF airways secretions, and the prevalence of obligate anaerobes is high among both children and adults with CF. Average colony counts of 5×10^7 bacteria/ml sputum demonstrate that the bacteria proliferate in the sputum, and are not simply the result of oral contamination. Up to half the strains tested are resistant to antibiotics that are frequently used in conventional CF therapy (e.g. ceftazidime), whereas the vast majority of the anaerobes are still susceptible to meropenem. Interestingly, half are also resistant to metronidazole, an antibiotic that is not usually employed in the treatment of CF lung infections.

The involvement of the obligate anaerobes in CF lung pathogenicity is still unclear. There is recent evidence that, in some patients, *Gemella* might play a direct role in and/or be a biomarker for pulmonary exacerbations. However, studies have not demonstrated a significant reduction of obligate anaerobic cell numbers or a change in community composition following treatment with antibiotics during exacerbations despite improvements in the patients' clinical status. At present, it is too early to make a recommendation for a specific therapy against the obligate anaerobes.

3.11 **Fungi**

3.11.1 *Aspergillus fumigatus*

Aspergillus fumigatus is the most common fungus isolated from CF respiratory tract samples. There are a number of manifestations of aspergillus disease in CF, including allergic bronchopulmonary aspergillosis (ABPA) and aspergillus bronchitis. The diagnosis of these different syndromes and the differentiation of aspergillus–related pathology from transient colonization and/or simple sensitisation can be challenging due to the overlap with symptoms and signs associated with other common complications of CF lung disease.

1. Allergic bronchopulmonary aspergillosis (ABPA) is an immune-mediated hypersensitivity response to antigens of aspergillus. Patients have raised aspergillus-specific skin-prick tests and/or IgE levels, have declining lung function and may often describe wheeziness and the expectoration of sputum plugs, and develop new radiographic features. Treatment is usually with oral corticosteroids, often with the addition of azoles to reduce fungal load and to act as steroid-sparing agents (see Chapter 4).

2. Aspergillus bronchitis has recently been recognized as a disease entity in CF patients who have aspergillus repeatedly isolated in sputum samples, declining lung function, and raised aspergillus-specific IgG antibody levels (though typically not with elevated IgE). Treatment is usually with azoles.

3. Aspergillomas. Although relatively rare in CF, when present, aspergillomas can pose problems particularly for patients at the time of lung transplantation.

3.11.2 **Other fungal species**

Candida albicans is also commonly isolated from respiratory tract secretions of CF patients, and whilst frequently considered as colonizer, it has been linked to risk of hospitalization and lower lung function. Other fungi including *Exophilala dermatidis* and *Scedosporium azospermum* are also encountered and have been associated with clinical decline in individual patients.

Dedication

The previous version of this chapter was co-authored by the late, sorely missed and much admired Professor Gerd Döring. In revising the chapter, the present authors have tried to retain as much as possible of Gerd's original themes and format. They are honoured to be able to dedicate their efforts to Gerd's memory.

References

Anstead M, Heltshe SL, Khan U. Pseudomonas aeruginosa serology and risk for re-isolation in the EPIC trial. *J Cyst Fibrosis* 2013;12:147–53.

Bartholdson SJ, Brown AR, Mewburn BR, et al. Plant host and sugar alcohol induced exopolysaccharide biosynthesis in the Burkholderia cepacia complex. *Microbiology* 2008;154:2513–21.

Bryant JM, Grogono DM, Greaves D, et al. Whole genome sequencing to identify transmission of Mycobacterium abscessus between patients with cystic fibrosis: a retrospective cohort study. *Lancet* 2013;381 (9877):1551–60

Döring G, Flume P, Heijerman H, et al. for the Consensus Study Group. Treatment of lung infection in patients with cystic fibrosis: current and future strategies. *J Cyst Fibrosis* 2012;11:461–79.

Döring G, Meisner C, Stern M. A double-blind randomized placebo-controlled phase III study of a Pseudomonas aeruginosa flagella vaccine in cystic fibrosis patients. *PNAS* 2007;104:11020–5.

Horsley A, Jones AM. Antibiotic treatment for Burkholderia cepacia complex in people with cystic fibrosis experiencing a pulmonary exacerbation. *Cochrane Database Syst Rev* 2012;Oct 17; CD009529.

Lipuma JJ. The changing microbial epidemiology in cystic fibrosis. *Clin Microbiol Rev* 2010;23:299–323.

Tunney MM, Field TR, Moriarty TF, et al. Detection of anaerobic bacteria in high numbers in sputum from patients with cystic fibrosis. *Am J Respir Crit Care Med* 2008;177:995–1001.

UK CF Trust Infection Control Working Group. *Methicillin resistant Staphylococcus aureus.* CF Trust, 2008.

UK CF Trust. *Laboratory standards for processing microbiological samples from people with cystic fibrosis.* CF Trust, 2010.

Zlosnik JEA, Hird TJ, Fraenkel MC, et al. Different mucoid exopolysaccahride production by members of the Burkholderia cepacia complex. *J Clin Microbiol* 2008;46:1470–3.

Chapter 4

Management of stable CF lung disease

Nicholas Simmonds and Elaine Dhouieb

Key points

- Aggressive treatment of specific lung infections improves prognosis
- Eradication of new *Pseudomonas* infection slows progression to chronic infection
- Effective airway clearance and mobilization of airway secretions is integral to improving outcomes
- Azithromycin, nebulized antibiotics, and mucolytic therapies can reduce the burden of infective exacerbations and improve lung function
- New mutation-specific therapies may modify disease and improve prognosis

4.1 Introduction

The progressive improvement in outlook for patients with CF in recent years reflects the adoption of a variety of proactive treatment strategies, which together maintain good lung health through childhood and well into adult life. A fundamental early step was the recognition by Canadian clinicians of the clear link between good nutritional status and lung health in cystic fibrosis. Nutritional therapy sufficient to normalize body mass index clearly improves lung function and is an important goal of effective CF care (see Chapter 7).

This chapter outlines the respiratory treatments which have contributed to improved prognosis. Pulmonary interventions capable of slowing the progress of lung disease have historically fallen into two main categories: those improving the clearance of infected sputum, and those directed primarily at reducing the burden of inflammation and infection in the CF lung. An important third category has recently been introduced, mutation specific therapy. This targets the basic cellular defect by modifying the function of the mutated CF protein (cystic fibrosis transmembrane conductance regulator or CFTR, see Chapter 1).

4.1.1 Clinical features

In early, mild disease, examination of the chest is normal. Cough is a prominent early symptom, and may lead to the false initial diagnosis of cough-variant asthma in a child. The cough is initially dry, but episodes of purulent sputum production soon supervene. Coarse crackles develop over the affected region and probably represent the presence of viscous secretions in small- and medium-sized airways. As time passes, features of chronic airflow obstruction develop, including a barrel-shaped chest, loss of cardiac dullness, reduced crico-sternal distance, and paradoxical inward movement of the lower ribs on inspiration (indicating a low, flat diaphragm). Coarse crackles become generalized, and areas of scarring, most common in the upper lobes, may lead to patches of bronchial breathing with increased vocal resonance. By this stage, accompanying finger clubbing is almost universal.

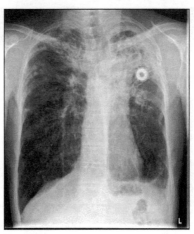

Figure 4.1 Chest X-ray in advanced CF. Note scarring and loss of volume in left upper lobe, also vascular access port on chest wall.

4.1.2 **Radiological features**

The chest radiograph is normal in early life. The earliest changes are usually streaky infil-trates in the upper lobes, which may initially clear between infections, but later become persistent. As bronchiectasis develops, ring shadows and 'tram line' parallel lines radiating from the hila (indicating thickened bronchial walls seen from the side) may appear, but these classical appearances are relatively uncommon and the plain radiograph is notoriously insensitive to early bronchiectatic change. In established CF lung disease (Figure 4.1), there are increased coarse lung makings in all lung fields. Scarring in the upper lobes frequently results in elevation of the hilar shadows.

Computed tomography (CT) is far more sensitive than plain radiographs for demonstrat-ing early bronchiectasis. Thick-walled airways are clearly seen, and CT also demonstrates mucus-filled bronchi and bronchioles (Figure 4.2), air trapping, and patchy infective infil-trates. CT is used increasingly to document and quantify the extent of CF lung disease, but radiation dose precludes routine serial use. CT is particularly useful if mycobacterial disease or aspergilloma is suspected.

4.2 **Physiotherapy**

Specialist physiotherapy input is essential in a variety of areas for the care of people with CF:

- Airway clearance techniques
- Devices for inhalation therapy
- Exercise
- Postural management

Physiotherapists are also involved in the management of specific issues such as musculoskel-etal problems, urinary continence (both covered in Chapter 9) and sinus disease.

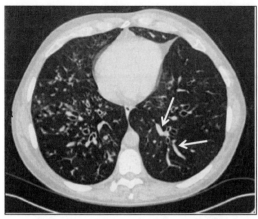

Figure 4.2 CT thorax in advanced CF. Note generalized thickening and dilation of the bronchi. Mucus-plugged airways are also seen in longitudinal section in the left lower lobe (arrows).

4.2.1 **Airway clearance techniques (ACT)**

Effective airway clearance can be achieved in a variety of ways. There is currently insufficient evidence to suggest superiority of any single technique. Selecting valid, reliable, and responsive outcome measures is challenging as infants and children often do not produce sputum and have normal chest radiography, clinical scores, and spirometry. ACT method selection should therefore be based on the patient's preference, circumstance, and clinical reasoning. Techniques may be combined depending on patient needs. Commonly used techniques are summarized in Table 4.1.

Once the appropriate ACT has been identified, it is important to coordinate the timing of inhaled medications around treatment sessions to ensure maximum benefit. Duration and frequency of ACT sessions will vary according to the patient's symptoms and lifestyle but some form of daily ACT is generally recommended in all patients.

4.2.2 **Devices for inhalation**

The choice of inhalation device for nebulized therapies is increasing all the time. Device selection, education, and provision, along with the initiation of new inhaled drugs, are often undertaken by a physiotherapist. The most common nebulizer devices are: conventional (compressed air) nebulization systems, ultrasonic nebulizers, adaptive aerosol delivery devices (AAD), and vibrating mesh technology systems (VMT). There is little evidence to recommend one type of nebulizer device over another in terms of clinical efficacy. New nebulizer technologies such as AAD and VMT have practical advantages over conventional systems as they are generally faster, quieter, and may have improved and more consistent lung deposition. Appropriate cleaning and maintenance of nebulizer equipment is essential to avoid bacterial contamination and to ensure efficiency of drug delivery. Dry powder inhalation is now available for some drugs. These devices are small, quiet, and quicker than nebulizers, and cleaning is not required. However, they are not suitable for everyone as a relatively high frequency of inhaler-associated cough has been reported and patients with severely impaired lung function may not be able to inspire the drug effectively.

Table 4.1 Summary of airway clearance techniques

Technique	Description	Comments
Positioning, percussion, and vibration, or 'conventional physiotherapy'	Positioning to change ventilation combined with chest percussion or vibration is used in babies and young children who are unable to alter volume and flow. This requires the caregiver to deliver treatment.	Gravity-assisted positions of postural drainage have largely fallen out of use due to the increased risk of gastro-oesophageal reflux and development of more active techniques. These techniques may not be appropriate in those with low mineral bone density.
Active cycle of breathing technique (ACBT)	This consists of using changes in volume and flow to move secretions and divert air into previously underventilated areas. It consists of a sequence of relaxed breathing control followed by 3–4 deep breaths for thoracic expansion then forced expirations or 'huffs'.	This may be performed independently in any position of comfort and may be combined with adjunct devices as described below. As it is not dependent on a device, it is one of the 2 airway clearance techniques, along with autogenic drainage, that every patient should be taught.
Autogenic drainage (AD)	Autogenic drainage is a 3-phased breathing regime using high expiratory flow rates at varying lung volumes to facilitate mucus clearance. The technique aims to maximize expiratory flow velocity to produce shearing forces and mobilise secretions. While expiratory flow should be high, it should not be forced (as this causes airway closure).	The avoidance of airway closure as described in AD may be beneficial particularly in patients with significant hyper-reactivity or unstable airways. This may be performed independently in any position of comfort and may be combined with adjunct devices as described below. Assisted AD can be used in infants and young children.
Positive expiratory pressure (PEP)	This is exhalation into a mask or mouthpiece providing a positive pressure, thus splinting open the smaller airways to avoid early closure and potential trapping of sputum. Periods of PEP breathing are combined with the active techniques above to facilitate airway clearance. PEP causes a temporary increase in functional residual capacity (FRC), increases interdependence between alveoli, facilitates collateral ventilatory flow, and therefore recruits previously closed airways.	It is suggested that the PEP-induced increase in gas volume and pressure behind airway secretions make expiratory manoeuvres more effective. The level of the expiratory resistor used should be regularly reassessed and may need to be changed with changes in clinical status.

Bubble PEP	This uses exactly the same action as PEP described above, but instead of using a mask or mouthpiece, the child blows out through a length of plastic tubing placed in a bottle of water and liquid soap to produce bubbles.	Bubble PEP is another modification of PEP and is very useful in young children. This is a fun way of getting small children to do PEP therapy.
Intra-thoracic oscillating positive expiratory pressure (OPEP)	These devices combine vibration of the airways with PEP. Exhalation into a hand-held device, such as the Flutter®, Acapella® or Cornet®, generates an oscillatory positive pressure. The vibratory effect is thought to reduce sputum viscosity. It may also improve airway patency by preventing spontaneous compression through the introduction of alternating positive pressure where the consequent vibration loosens mucus allowing ease of expectoration.	The Flutter is gravity-dependent and only functions in the upright position whereas the Acapella and Cornet may be used in any position of comfort. Intrapulmonary percussive vibration (IPV) may also be used in some centres.
Extra-thoracic oscillations (high-frequency chest wall oscillation, HFCWO) 'The Vest'	A mechanical device consisting of an inflatable jacket and air pulse generator that produces chest wall oscillation.	Less common in UK compared to USA due to high costs and limited evidence base. A recent well conducted long-term study showed no long-term benefit.
Non-invasive ventilation (NIV)	NIV may be useful as an adjunct to ACT but there is a lack of robust evidence to support its use. May be used to reduce the work of ACT.	Effective airway clearance techniques may be challenging for some patients with advanced disease due to increased ventilatory demand, alterations in gas exchange and dyspnoea.

4.2.3 **Exercise**

Exercise has been linked to improved survival in CF and is associated with other benefits: a reduction in loss of bone mineral density, maintenance of chest wall mobility, and better self-esteem. There is also some evidence that it may enhance sputum clearance. Current general guidelines for physical activity for healthy children and adults are also applicable in CF and can be used as a basis for exercise advice until respiratory disease progresses. Advice, education, and motivation to be active should start from diagnosis and reviewed regularly. Formal cardiopulmonary exercise testing may help target more prescriptive activities for patients who are either deconditioned or have ventilatory limitation.

4.2.4 **Postural management**

Poor posture and flexibility are common features in patients with CF. CF-related bone disease and abnormal respiratory mechanics lead to a high incidence of musculoskeletal pain, thoracic kyphosis, and vertebral fracture rates. All patients should have an annual musculoskeletal and postural assessment from childhood (age ~8 years), with monitoring and treatment of any musculoskeletal issues (see Chapter 9).

4.3 **Drugs to aid secretion clearance**

There is good evidence to support the use of 3 different drugs to treat sputum and aid airway clearance in CF: recombinant dornase alfa, hypertonic saline, and mannitol. No trial has been conducted that has definitively shown superiority of one over the other, and some trials include dornase alfa as standard of care. It is therefore important to tailor the treatment to the individual based on their clinical response, and to consider adding a therapy if there is evidence of accelerated decline or symptomatic difficulty expectorating.

4.3.1 **Recombinant dornase alfa**

The high viscosity of sputum in CF is believed to result in large part from the DNA released from dead neutrophils. Recombinant human dornase alfa liquefies sputum *in vitro* by digesting the extracellular DNA molecules into smaller nucleotide chains. It is available as unit dose vials of 2.5 mg for once-daily nebulized administration. Several randomized controlled trials have demonstrated, in large numbers of patients, a mean improvement in FEV_1 of around 9% at 1 month, falling to 5% at 6 months. Some trials suggest a trend to reduced frequency of exacerbations in treated patients. The benefits are less clear in patients with severe lung disease (FVC <40% predicted) although registry data suggest a benefit does exist.

In practice, individual response is variable, with some patients gaining clear clinical benefit and others noticing no change. Because response is unpredictable, patients with productive cough or lung function decline are commonly given a trial period of dornase alfa treatment (up to 6 months) after which they agree with their physician whether or not the benefits (based on lung function and symptoms) warrant continuation.

4.3.2 **Hypertonic saline**

Hypertonic saline (HS) is administered by nebulizer with the aim of increasing the osmotic pressure of the airway-lining fluid, drawing water into the airway. Early studies confirmed improved mucociliary clearance, though HS can cause cough and bronchospasm. A large controlled trial of HS (4 ml of 7% NaCl nebulized twice a day over 48 weeks) showed only modest effects on FEV_1 (3.2% rise), but a reduction in the number of exacerbations and the number of days with exacerbation symptoms. A bronchodilator was used routinely prior to HS administration to prevent bronchospasm, but cough was still a significant adverse effect with HS treatment.

4.3.3 **Mannitol**

Mannitol is a naturally occurring sugar found in most plants. Like hypertonic saline it is a hyperosmotic agent and functions by drawing water onto the airway lining to improve sputum clearance. It has been developed as a dry powder and therefore can be administered using an inhalation device, making administration and delivery more convenient for most users. Two large randomized controlled trials of dry powder mannitol have shown benefit with pooled data demonstrating a modest relative improvement in FEV_1 of 3.6%, (only statistically significant for adults). A significant reduction in pulmonary exacerbations of 29% was demonstrated. Similar to hypertonic saline, cough and bronchoconstriction can occur, so careful education of administration technique and monitoring of spirometry during an initiation test is important.

4.3.4 **Other therapies**

The maintenance of adequate systemic hydration is considered important as it probably facilitates the hydration of airway secretions and sputum clearance. Patients who are systemically unwell, especially if pyrexial, should therefore be considered for IV fluids and humidified oxygen therapy if hypoxic (see Chapter 5).

The use of oral or nebulized thiol derivatives (e.g. N-acetylcysteine or carbocysteine) as a mucolytic agent in CF is of no proven benefit. A recent Cochrane review concluded that although the drugs were well tolerated, there was no evidence of significant clinical benefit.

4.4 **Airway infection and inflammation**

4.4.1 **Inhaled antibiotics**

For CF patients with chronic airway infection with *Pseudomonas aeruginosa*, nebulized antibiotics have been used for many years, particularly in Europe. The polymyxin antibiotic colistimethate sodium is widely used in the UK by inhalation (see Chapter 14 for dosing). Although studies have demonstrated a reduction in sputum bacterial load and improved symptom scores, large randomized trials showing functional improvement (e.g. improved lung function or reduced exacerbation rate) are lacking.

Nebulized aminoglycosides have also been used in CF patients for many years, and a formulation of tobramycin specifically for nebulized use was tested against placebo in a large randomized US trial published in 1999. Tobramycin given 300 mg bd by nebulizer during alternate months increased lung function, and reduced hospitalization rates and the need for intravenous antibiotics compared to placebo. The medication was well tolerated and resistance to tobramycin did not appear to limit clinical efficacy.

More recently, the monobactam antibiotic, aztreonam, has been developed for inhalation as nebulized aztreonam lysine. It is used to treat chronic *P. aeruginosa* infection and is administered during alternate months at a dose of 75 mg three times daily.

With the exception of colistimethate sodium, inhaled antibiotics have been developed and licensed for alternate-month administration to reduce the theoretical risk of bacterial resistance. The disadvantage of this is that patients often feel worse during the month with no antibiotic cover, so monthly alternating antibiotic strategies (e.g. colistimethate sodium alternating with tobramycin) are often recommended to provide more effective continuous cover.

The antibiotics armoury has recently widened further with the introduction of dry powder inhalers for colistimethate sodium and tobramycin. These devices are generally easy to use and more convenient than nebulizers because they do not require cleaning and tend to have a faster administration time. Clinical trials have demonstrated non-inferiority to tobramycin nebulizer solution for both.

For particularly resistant bacteria, such as *Burkholderia cepacia* complex and *Mycobacterium abscessus*, treatment options are limited and therefore other, non-licensed, nebulized treatments are sometimes used with careful monitoring, including meropenem, ceftazidime, and amikacin.

Recommendations

- In the UK, patients with chronic *P. aeruginosa* infection are usually offered nebulized colistimethate sodium 2 MU bd (1 MU bd for children) as first-line treatment
- Nebulized tobramycin 300 mg bd alternate months is used for patients who are intolerant of colistimethate sodium and those whose clinical condition deteriorates while receiving colistimethate sodium (i.e. second-line). Nebulized aztreonam lysine 75 mg tds is used for patients who are intolerant of colistimethate sodium and/or tobramycin or those whose clinical condition deteriorates while receiving tobramycin (i.e. third-line)
- It may be appropriate to use continuous monthly alternating antibiotics for sustained bacterial suppression, especially if a patient demonstrates evidence of clinical decline when not covered by an antibiotic
- Inhaled antibiotics are now available as a dry powder or nebulizer solution—selection is based on patient choice and local/national guidelines
- The first dose of a nebulized or dry powder antibiotic should be given under appropriate supervision with spirometry pre and post dosing in order to monitor for bronchoconstriction

4.4.2 **Oral macrolides**

The striking efficacy of erythromycin in bronchiectasis associated with Japanese panbronchiolitis prompted several large controlled trials of oral macrolides in CF. The precise mechanism of action of macrolides in bronchiectasis remains unclear. In stable laboratory cultures (as opposed to exponential growth cultures), macrolides appear to have bactericidal effects on *P. aeruginosa*. In addition, *in vitro* studies have demonstrated that macrolides can suppress pro-inflammatory cytokines and modulate neutrophil function.

A large randomized placebo-controlled trial of azithromycin (500 mg oral 3 times a week; 250 mg if <40 kg) in *Pseudomonas*-infected CF patients demonstrated a modest mean improvement in lung function but a significantly reduced risk of a pulmonary exacerbation compared to placebo, over the 6-month trial period. A further large placebo-controlled trial extended these observations in a group of children, most of whom were not infected with *P. aeruginosa*. In this year-long study, a significant reduction in exacerbation rate was demonstrated.

This chronic oral treatment, normally given 3 times a week, is popular with patients as it is quick and convenient to take, and free of major side effects.

Recommendations

- Regular oral macrolides (e.g. azithromycin 500 mg three times a week (250 mg if <40 kg)) should be considered in all patients infected with *P.aeruginosa*, particularly those deteriorating on conventional therapy, although they should be withheld in patients with non-tuberculous mycobacterial infection to preserve their antimycobacterial activity
- Evidence of benefit in those without *P. aeruginosa* is less strong, however a trial of treatment is reasonable in those with frequent chest exacerbations

4.4.3 **Inhaled steroids**

The role of inhaled steroids in cystic fibrosis lung disease is contentious. The predominantly neutrophil-mediated inflammation in the airways of CF patients is believed to contribute to progressive damage to the airways over time, and oral corticosteroids may reduce the progression of lung disease. The long-term use of oral steroids is, however, precluded by adverse effects, particularly on skin, glucose tolerance, bone density, and (in children) on growth.

Given the existing widespread use of inhaled steroids in CF, prospective trials of their effects are impractical to perform. A large multicentre randomized controlled trial of withdrawal of established inhaled steroid treatment, however, showed that most patients receiving this treatment can stop it without any detectable decline in lung function or increased risk of exacerbation of their chest disease. Thus, while there may be a small subgroup of patients with coincident asthma who do benefit from inhaled steroids, generalized prescription of these drugs to all CF patients is not supported by the evidence.

4.4.4 Other therapies

Flucloxacillin

Pulmonary infection with *Staphylococcus aureus* is a frequent problem in patients with CF, particularly during the first decade of life (see Chapter 3). Although the pathogen is frequently associated with an increase in symptoms, its effect on lung function and survival has never been fully established. As no randomized controlled trials with the anti-staphylococcal antibiotic, flucloxacillin, have been conducted, efficacy has never been proven. For these reasons treatment strategies are inconsistent, from commencement at CF diagnosis as a preventative strategy, to intercurrent short courses when it is isolated from the respiratory tract. Early and continuous use of anti-staphylococcal antibiotics has raised concerns over the development of resistant strains and earlier acquisition of *P. aeruginosa* (with cefalexin), but further prospective studies are required to substantiate these.

Vaccination

Annual influenza vaccination should be offered routinely to all patients with established CF lung disease, because influenza may be associated with severe pulmonary exacerbations.

4.5 Mutation-specific therapies

An exciting new area of drug development in CF is mutation-specific therapy. Until now, the mainstay of drug treatment has focused on minimizing the cycle of injury by treating airway infection and mucus accumulation. These therapies are treating pathophysiological consequences of CFTR dysfunction and may be too late to modulate the disease process. Therapies aimed at early steps are more likely to halt disease progression and ultimately to improve the quality and length of life. A number of products are under development and some have progressed to phase 3 clinical trials (see Chapter 13). One product, ivacaftor, has been approved by European and US regulators and is available to patients. Ivacaftor is administered as a twice-daily tablet of 150 mg (adults) and is indicated for patients with the specific class 3 mutation, *G551D* (see Chapter 1). It works by potentiating the function of the faulty CFTR protein, allowing chloride to flow out of cells more effectively, thus improving the ion transport and electrophysiological deficits of CF. In clinical trials, patients with at least one *G551D* mutation had a 10% increase in percent of predicted FEV_1. Other benefits included a reduction in pulmonary exacerbations, an improvement in weight, and a reduction in sweat chloride, suggesting widespread CFTR modulation.

4.6 Specific complications of CF lung disease

4.6.1 New sputum isolation of *Pseudomonas aeruginosa*

Patients with airway infection caused by *Pseudomonas* have a more rapid decline in lung function and chest X-ray scores, need more hospital days and courses of antibiotics, and

> **Box 4.1 Eradication of** *P. aeruginosa*
>
> • Nebulized colistimethate sodium 1 MU (<2 yrs) or 2 MU (>2 yrs) 8–12 hrly
>
> AND
>
> • Oral ciprofloxacin: 15 mg/kg (<5 yrs) / 20 mg/kg (>5 yrs) / 750 mg (adults) every 12 hrs
>
> for 3 months
>
> Inhaled tobramycin may be used in those showing early regrowth of *Pseudomonas*, or if intolerant of ciprofloxacin or colistimethate sodium.

suffer impaired growth compared to matched controls without this common CF pathogen. Studies in this area are plagued by the difficulty in distinguishing between the effects of the organism itself and its presence simply reflecting a more severe lung phenotype. Standard clinical practice, however, is to make aggressive efforts with anti-pseudomonal antibiotics to eradicate *P. aeruginosa* following first isolation (see Chapter 3).

There are a number of small controlled clinical trials which confirm that it is possible using oral quinolones and/or inhaled tobramycin or colistimethate sodium to eradicate *P. aeruginosa* from recently infected patients. The UK CF Trust recommends oral ciprofloxacin and nebulized colistimethate sodium for up to 3 months as primary eradication treatment following first *P. aeruginosa* isolation (Box 4.1). Recent evidence from a multicentre randomized controlled trial has shown a 1-month course of single-agent nebulized tobramycin is also an effective eradication strategy. Newer inhaled preparations of colistimethate sodium and tobramycin have not been assessed for this indication, but are expected to be an equally effective alternative. If *P. aeruginosa* persists despite oral ± nebulized antibiotic strategies, most centres follow this with intravenous anti-pseudomonal antibiotics. With these, *P. aeruginosa* can be eradicated in the majority of cases, and it is now increasingly common for adolescent CF patients to undergo transition to adult services without chronic *P. aeruginosa* airway infection.

4.6.2 *Aspergillus* in CF

Airway colonization by the environmental fungus *Aspergillus fumigatus* is very common in CF. In most cases, *Aspergillus* appears to colonize the airways without causing harm, at least in earlier stages. A proportion of patients, however, develop allergy to *Aspergillus* with high blood levels of specific IgE, *Aspergillus* precipitins, and eosinophilia. This may be associated with new X-ray infiltrates and worsening chest symptoms. As with allergic bronchopulmonary aspergillosis (ABPA) in asthma patients, treatment is directed at suppressing allergy using oral steroids and suppressing the organism with antifungal agents. Triazoles (particularly itraconazole) are commonly used in combination with prednisolone. Case reports suggest that the anti-IgE antibody omalizumab may have useful steroid-sparing benefits in CF patients with ABPA.

Diagnosis of ABPA

Diagnosis relies on a combination of the following criteria. Note that IgE levels may be affected by systemic steroids and cutaneous reactivity by antihistamines.

• Acute or subacute clinical deterioration, not due to another cause

• Serum IgE >500 IU/ml

• Skin prick positive to *Aspergillus* antigens, or *in vitro* demonstration of
  Aspergillus-specific IgE

AND at least one of:

- *Aspergillus* precipitins or specific IgG
- New or recent infiltrates or mucus plugging on CXR or CT, not responding to conventional therapy

Recommendations

- Standard initial treatment for symptomatic patients with proven ABPA and CF is prednisolone (0.5–1 mg/kg/d, maximum 60 mg) together with itraconazole. Prolonged therapy (months) is usually required to control symptoms. The dose is reduced after the first 1–2 weeks, and then tapered to the lowest possible, to minimize side effects
- Patients starting itraconazole should have liver function tests checked at the start of therapy, after 1 month, then 3 monthly

In addition to ABPA, other responses to *Aspergillus* in the CF lung are now recognized, including infection with lung function decline but without evidence of allergic mediation, for which the term '*aspergillus* bronchitis' is sometimes used. Optimal treatment strategies are not known but probably include prolonged triazole courses.

4.6.3 **Sinonasal disease**

The electrophysiological defect of CF affects the entire respiratory epithelium, including the lining of the nose and nasal sinuses. Common manifestations of CF in the upper airway include nasal polyps and chronic sinusitis. Patients may present with symptoms of nasal obstruction, anosmia, persistent purulent discharge, or facial pain from sinus infection and obstructed drainage. For lesser degrees of nasal obstruction, nasal steroid sprays are often sufficient. Nasal douching with saline or sodium bicarbonate can be used to aid clearance of sinus and nasal secretions. Polyps may be large in which case ENT referral for surgical resection is usually indicated.

Infective sinusitis may cause severe pain and require intravenous antibiotic treatment. Surgical sinus drainage procedures occasionally help those with recurrent symptoms, although these are rarely a permanent solution and the problem typically recurs. Sinus problems persist following lung transplantation; indeed transplant immunosuppression may exacerbate the problem so patients newly free of lower respiratory problems may still be burdened with the need for intravenous antibiotics.

4.7 **Travel considerations**

Improvements in the health status of individuals with CF over the past few decades have enabled them to participate in every aspect of modern life, including travel and tourism. This should be respected and supported in most situations, however, careful preparation before traveling is important. Obtaining appropriate medical insurance, vaccinations, and letters to validate the need to travel with drugs and equipment (e.g. nebulizers) are important. Before holidays are even booked patients should be made aware of areas to avoid including Southeast Asia and northern Australia due to the prevalence of the highly pathogenic organism *Burkholderia pseudomallei*. Specific activities should be avoided, including scuba diving (risk of pneumothorax) and the use of jacuzzis (which may harbor potentially harmful pathogens, such as *P. aeruginosa*). Considerations for continuing treatments, including physiotherapy, and drug storage (e.g. refrigeration for dornase alfa) should be made. Counselling should be provided for the appropriate use of salt tablets and maintaining hydration in hot climates. If air travel is planned, the duration of the flight and patient condition are the main predictors of medical safety during air travel. Prediction of in-flight oxygen using British Thoracic Society guidelines (2002) should be used, especially in individuals with moderate to severe lung disease (FEV$_1$ <55% predicted, resting SpO2 <95% on air) or a pre-existing requirement for supplementary oxygen. An awareness of the country of destination's healthcare infrastructure and contacts for CF-specific care, if available, is also recommended.

References

ACPCF Standards of Care and Good Clinical Practice for the Physiotherapy Management of Cystic Fibrosis. CF Trust, 2011.

Bilton D, Robinson P, Cooper P, et al. Inhaled dry powder mannitol in cystic fibrosis: an efficacy and safety study. *European Respiratory Journal* 2011;38:1071–80.

CF Trust Antibiotic Working Group. *Antibiotic Treatment for Cystic Fibrosis.* CF Trust. May 2009.

Elkins MR, Robinson M, Rose BR, et al. A Controlled Trial of Long-Term Inhaled Hypertonic Saline in Patients with Cystic Fibrosis. *N Eng J Med* 2006;354:229–240.

International Physiotherapy Group for Cystic Fibrosis IPG/CF. Physiotherapy for people with Cystic Fibrosis: from infant to adult. 2009.

Jones AP, Wallis CE. Dornase alfa for cystic fibrosis. *Cochrane Database Syst Rev* 2010;(3):CD001127.

Ramsey BW, Davies J, McElvaney NG, et al. A CFTR potentiator in patients with cystic fibrosis and the G551D mutation. *N Eng J Med* 2011;365:1663–72.

Ramsey BW, Pepe MS, Quan JM, et al. Intermittent administration of inhaled tobramycin in patients with cystic fibrosis. *N Eng J Med* 1999;340:23–30.

Saiman L, Marshall BC, Mayer-Hablett N, et al. Azithromycin in patients with cystic fibrosis chronically infected with Pseudomonas aeruginosa: a randomized controlled trial. *JAMA* 2003;290:1749–56.

Chapter 5

Management of respiratory exacerbations

Francis J Gilchrist and Alex Horsley

> **Key points**
>
> - Early recognition and treatment of CF exacerbations is one of the cornerstones of CF care
> - Diagnosis is essentially clinical, based on patient symptoms and baseline investigations
> - Mild exacerbations are usually treated with oral antibiotics and more severe exacerbations with intravenous antibiotics
> - The choice of antibiotic is guided by the organisms regularly cultured from the patient, the antimicrobial sensitivities, the presence of antibiotic intolerance/ allergy, and the previous responses to treatment
> - In patients with chronic *Pseudomonas aeruginosa* infection, a combination of a β-lactam and an aminoglycoside antibiotic is usually used. Monotherapy should be avoided
> - There is a lack of evidence regarding the duration of treatment. Most clinicians use 14 days but this may be altered according to the clinical response
> - Antibiotics may need to be changed if the patient is not responding to treatment or a new organism is identified
> - Treatment can be delivered at home but requires the same assessment and monitoring that inpatients receive
> - Treatment is multidisciplinary and also involves attention to physiotherapy, nutrition, and glucose homeostasis

5.1 Presentation and assessment

CF lung disease is characterized by a vicious cycle of infection, inflammation, and lung damage, resulting in a progressive loss of lung function. In addition to daily symptoms such as cough and sputum production, patients are likely to be affected by recurrent episodes of increased pulmonary symptoms, termed exacerbations. These episodes are important events in the natural history of CF as they are associated with a more rapid deterioration in lung function, poorer quality of lif,e and higher mortality. In addition to this burden on the patient there is a significant financial burden associated with the cost of antibiotic treatment and hospitalization. The prevention of pulmonary exacerbations is one of the main outcome measures used to measure the success of chronic CF treatments. Despite the importance of pulmonary exacerbations in CF, there is general paucity of evidence regarding their treatment. Most guidelines have to rely on consensus statements rather than data from clinical trials.

5.1.1 **Diagnosis**

Despite the central role of exacerbations in the clinical course of CF, there is no universally agreed definition of what constitutes an exacerbation. In research studies, a number of different scoring systems have been devised that combine patient symptoms with clinical evaluation and data from laboratory and lung function assessments.

In the absence of an agreed definition, the diagnosis of a CF respiratory exacerbation remains essentially clinical, and typically relies on the presence of a number of the signs and symptoms listed in Table 5.1. These symptoms and signs can be respiratory-specific

Table 5.1 Signs and symptoms associated with pulmonary exacerbation
Pulmonary signs and symptoms (new or increased)
Exertional dyspnoea or reduced exercise tolerance*
Cough*
Wheeze

Change in sputum production:
   Volume*
   Appearance
   Colour (usually darker)*
   Consistency (usually thicker)*

Haemoptysis
Increased respiratory rate*

Change in respiratory examination*
   Recession or use of accessory muscles
   Change in chest sounds

Decreased lung function   Fall in FEV_1 by ≥10% over usual baseline
Upper respiratory tract symptoms
Sore throat/coryza
Sinus pain or tenderness
Change in sinus discharge
Constitutional signs and symptoms
Malaise/fatigue
Fever
Decreased appetite/anorexia*
Weight loss*
Work/school absenteeism
Investigations
New CXR changes
Reduced oxygen saturations
Increase peripheral blood neutrophil count ($\geq 15 \times 10^9 l^{-1}$)

Those indicated by a * are those most strongly associated with a diagnosis of exacerbation.

Reprinted from J. Pediatr., 148 /2, Ferkol T., Cystic fibrosis pulmonary exacerbations, 259–264, Copyright (2006), with permission from Elsevier.

(increased cough, change in sputum volume, colour, or consistency, increased respiratory rate, new examination findings, or reduced spirometry), or non-specific and systemic (decreased appetite, weight loss, and lethargy). In the absence of symptoms, isolated changes in lung function, radiology, or laboratory findings should prompt further evaluation to identify the cause. The diagnosis of exacerbations is more difficult in young children as typically they do not produce sputum or perform spirometry (both easily quantifiable). The diagnosis therefore relies on more subjective features such as constitutional upset, parent report of cough, failure to gain weight, and the development of new respiratory signs.

5.1.2 **Assessment of severity**

The decision to use oral or intravenous antibiotics and the possible need for hospitalization is dependent on the severity of the exacerbation. This can vary from mild to life-threatening. Assessing the severity of an exacerbation is easier at the extremes but can be difficult as there is no definition for the severity of CF pulmonary exacerbations. Clinicians therefore rely on patient- or parent-reported outcomes, lung function results, and the effect that symptoms are having on the patient's quality of life or ability to perform normal activities. Box 5.1 lists the typical assessments that a patient will need before starting intravenous antibiotics.

5.1.3 **Pathophysiology**

Little is known about the underlying pathophysiology of pulmonary exacerbations in CF. Previously it was assumed that they were caused by the acquisition of a new organism or a progression of chronic infection and inflammation causing an increased bacterial burden. This bacterial burden was assumed to decrease with antibiotic use. Recent studies using culture-independent techniques have shown that the pathophysiology is far more complex and is likely to involve a web of interactions between anaerobic bacteria, aerobic bacteria, and viruses. Interestingly, although the composition of the CF lung microbiome varies between patients, it remains relatively stable during exacerbations and antibiotic treatment only causes a transient decrease in bacterial abundance.

Box 5.1 Assessment of patient

In patients being evaluated for intravenous antibiotics, the following assessments are recommended.
Full clinical exam, paying particular attention to:
  temperature
  respiratory rate
  oxygen saturations
  evidence of increased respiratory effort in young children
Sputum microbiology, or cough swab if not producing sputum (see Chapter 3)
Spirometry
Blood tests, including full blood count, electrolytes, liver function, CRP, and blood glucose
Chest X-ray if:
  suspected pneumothorax
  suspected lung collapse/consolidation
  disproportionate breathlessness or hypoxia
  failure to respond to therapy
Consider ABG/CBG in advanced disease to exclude CO_2 retention

In young children and infants, it may not be possible to perform lung function assessments, and chest X-ray is not usually indicated in most exacerbations

5.1.4 **Epidemiology of exacerbations**

The frequency of exacerbations increases with age and deteriorating lung function. On average, 23% of children under 6 years experience at least 1 exacerbation per year. This increases to 63% for patients over 18 years. Other factors associated with an increased frequency of exacerbations include infection with *Pseudomonas aeruginosa* (*Pa*), reactive airway disease, viral infections, lower socioeconomic status, and air pollution.

5.2 **Treatment of a pulmonary exacerbation**

5.2.1 **Principles of treatment**

There is a lack of randomized controlled clinical trials to guide treatment of exacerbations, but the following principles are generally applied:

1) Antibiotics are the mainstay of treatment

2) Patients chronic daily therapies such as nebulized mucolytics, airway clearance techniques, and CF-related diabetes treatment should be intensified/optimized

A number of questions need to be addressed regarding the use of antibiotics. These include:

1) Oral or intravenous?

2) Inpatient or outpatient?

3) Which antibiotic to use?

4) Duration of treatment?

The answers to these questions will be guided by the severity of the exacerbation but also by the patient history including response to previous exacerbations, any history of antibiotic hypersensitivity reactions, and the presence of comorbidities. Psychosocial factors such as adherence to treatment, motivation, and home situation are also important.

5.2.2 **Routes of delivery**

Antibiotics can be given orally, intravenously, or nebulized. Oral antibiotics are reserved for milder exacerbations when there is little constitutional upset, and for infections identified on surveillance cultures in the absence of symptoms. More serious exacerbations are treated with intravenous antibiotics. Nebulized antibiotics are used as part of the eradication regimen for *Pa* when first isolated (see Chapter 4), and as maintenance therapy in patients chronically infected *Pa* or *Burkholderia cepacia* complex (BCC). Their role in the treatment of acute exacerbations is less clear, but at present they are not usually employed in this role. Regular nebulized antibiotics should be continued whilst on IV antibiotics. Care must be taken when the nebulized drug is also prescribed for IV treatment (e.g. tobramycin) as this can lead to drug accumulation and toxicity. In such cases, plasma drug concentrations should be monitored more closely or the nebulized treatment discontinued for the duration of the intravenous treatment.

5.2.3 **Home treatment**

Most courses of oral antibiotic are given at home. Traditionally, treatment with intravenous antibiotics required hospitalization but more recently, home intravenous antibiotic treatment (HIVAT) has been shown to be a practical and effective alternative to inpatient administration. Providing patients are appropriately selected, HIVAT is as effective as inpatient treatment and in addition, it reduces disruption for patients and families, decreases the opportunity for cross-infection, and reduces costs. There is an added burden on the patient or parent, who must be taught to administer the antibiotics themselves (typically requiring 2–3 days of in patient education), and then prepare and administer the antibiotics (usually 2–4 different doses per day). It is important that patients on HIVAT are monitored to ensure response to the treatment. As a minimum, lung function and weight should be undertaken at the start, mid-point and end of the course. If the patient is not improving as expected, then the patient should be admitted for the remainder of their treatment. Contra-indications to HIVAT include the patient being too unwell or fatigued to administer the antibiotics or undertake their chronic daily therapies, lack of motivation, poor adherence to treatment, and poor social circumstances.

Recommendations

- Patients/carers must have previously undergone training in HIVAT, and be competent to carry it out. If not previously taught, a 2–3 day admission for intensive education and supervision is required.
- Prior to commencing HIVAT baseline height, weight, and lung function should be measured. Baseline bloods including FBC and CRP may also be taken.
- Administration of HIVAT is either via a totally indwelling venous access device (TIVAD) or a PICC line (see section 5.4).
- The first dose should be given under supervision in the unit and the patient monitored for the development of a hypersensitivity reaction for at least 60 minutes. If the patient has not previously received the antibiotic, he/she should be monitored as an inpatient for the first 1–2 days of treatment.
- Patients/carers should be provided with an anaphylaxis kit, and given clear written instructions in case of adverse reaction.
- Patients may need serum drug levels. Care needs to be taken to ensure these are taken at the correct time, the results noted, and any changes to the antibiotic doses communicated to the patient in a timely manner.
- Lung function and weight should be repeated after 7 days to assess response. Bloods may also be repeated. This can be done during a home visit or a hospital attendance.
- If the patient is not improving, or adherence is poor, he/she should be admitted for the remainder of the antibiotic course.
- At the end of the HIVAT course, patients need repeat measurements of weight and lung function and once the decision has been made to stop treatment, the lines can be removed.

5.2.4 **Identification of infecting organism**

It is important to have up-to-date culture results from the respiratory tract in order to guide appropriate antibiotic selection and to monitor for new infections. During the early stages of infection, patients are often asymptomatic so microbiology samples must be obtained routinely rather than waiting for symptoms to start. The gold-standard microbiology sample for patients with CF is expectorated sputum. Unfortunately, most young children and a significant proportion of adults are unable or unwilling to expectorate sputum. In these cases, the microbiological sample most commonly used is the orophayngeal 'cough' swab which is not as sensitive as expectorated sputum. If serial cough swabs remain negative when infection is suspected, other methods for sampling the respiratory tract may be undertaken such as flexible bronchoscopy with bronchoalveolar lavage, or the induction of sputum expectoration with nebulized hypertonic saline.

Recommendation

Appropriate cultures should be obtained at every clinic visit and prior to starting antibiotics.

5.2.5 **Duration of antibiotic therapy**

There is no clear evidence for the optimal duration of intravenous antibiotic therapy for the treatment of pulmonary exacerbations. Reviews of CF practice show that most courses of antibiotics are given for around 14 days and clinicians then use clinical parameters to increase or decrease the duration as appropriate. Successful treatment of an exacerbation is suggested by the reduction of symptoms to baseline levels and restoration of lung function. There is evidence that lung function frequently fails to return to pre-exacerbation levels despite treatment.

5.2.6 Elective versus symptomatic treatment

Some units apply a policy of regular (elective) antibiotic treatment (usually 3–6 monthly), irrespective of clinical condition. The rationale is that this reduces the bacteriological burden in the lung, which then reduces exacerbations and need for unplanned therapy. There is a theoretical risk of increased resistance if antibiotics are given more frequently. Studies on this are limited, but there is no evidence of a difference in clinical outcomes between elective and symptomatic antibiotics. In the absence of evidence, the decision to employ the elective approach is down to patient preference, and may be useful in those with frequent exacerbations or complex social circumstances.

An alternative use of elective antibiotics is immediately before events that are important to the patient (e.g. holidays, exams). This helps to avoid untimely therapy and ensure that they remain well for the event.

5.3 Antibiotic selection

5.3.1 Principles

Antibiotics are the mainstay of pulmonary exacerbation treatment and are usually selected according to the chronic bacterial infections identified in sputum cultures. This assumes that the patient's chronic infection is the cause of the acute exacerbation, or that when there is another cause (new bacteria or virus), the suppression of these bacteria will still be beneficial. In patients with no previously identified chronic bacterial infection, antibiotics must be chosen to target likely causative species.

Antibiotic choice may be guided by antimicrobial testing, but there is often discordance between the *in-vitro* test results and the clinical outcomes. This means that demonstrating resistance in the laboratory does not necessarily mean that the antibiotic will be ineffective when given to the patient. Antibiotic choice should, therefore, also be guided by previously effective treatments.

Treatment of exacerbations by *Pseudomonas* should involve the use of more than one antibiotic to reduce the development of bacterial resistance. The selected antibiotics should have different modes of action, e.g. a β-lactam and an aminoglycoside. There is no evidence to support routinely selecting antibiotics according to synergy testing.

The antibiotics chosen may need to be changed if a new infection is identified or if the clinical response to treatment is poor. Some examples of antibiotic regimens are given in section 5.3.

5.3.2 Pitfalls of antibiotic use in CF

Metabolism and clearance of some antibiotics is altered in CF, and the doses required to achieve therapeutic plasma levels are different from non-CF patients (see Chapter 14). Repeated dosing can lead to cumulative toxic effects (e.g. renal function and hearing impairment with aminoglycosides), and to the development of hypersensitivity. This must be balanced against evidence showing that more aggressive and early use of antibiotics results in better preservation of lung function. Gentamicin is no longer recommended in CF because of its association with renal failure. Tobramycin is the preferred aminoglycoside.

There is uncertainty as to the optimal antibiotic regime at different stages of CF lung disease, and local guidelines may differ. The primary aims are to select the most effective and least toxic regimen, and the secondary aims are to choose the most cost-effective treatment and avoid the development of antibiotic resistance. Table 5.2 shows the typical antibiotic sensitivities of the common infecting organisms in CF. The choice of antibiotics will depend on the known, and likely, infecting organisms, and the clinical severity of the infection.

5.3.3 Suggested antibiotic regimens

Non-Pseudomonas aeruginosa exacerbations

Non-*Pa* exacerbations are more common in children but also occur in a significant proportion of adults. For patients who have never cultured *Pa*, or who have had repeated negative cultures for over 12 months following *Pa* eradication therapy, a suggested approach to antibiotic selection is given in Figure 5.1.

The presence of *Pa* should be suspected in patients who have failed to respond well to 2 courses of non-*Pa* therapy, or in whom there has been a recent clinical deterioration. A concerted effort to obtain relevant airway cultures is necessary in these cases. In non-expectorating patients, an induced sputum or bronchoalveolar lavage may be indicated.

Exacerbation in patients with chronic Pseudomonas aeruginosa *infection*

Chronic *Pa* infection is common in older children and adults. Most will already be receiving long-term treatment with a nebulized anti-*Pa* antibiotic. Intravenous antibiotic monotherapy for *Pa* may encourage resistance and is therefore avoided. A suggested approach is illustrated in Figure 5.2.

Table 5.2 Antibiotic spectrum of activity					
Type	**Antibiotic**	**Cover**			
		SA	**HI**	**Pa**	**BCC**
β-lactam penicillin	Flucloxacillin	++	−	−	−
	Amoxicillin	−	+	−	−
	Co-amoxiclav	+	++	−	−
Cephalosporin	Cefuroxime	++	++	−	−
	Cefotaxime	+	++	−	−
	Ceftazidime	−	++	++	+
Fluroquinolone	Ciprofloxacin	+	++	++	−
Anti-pseudomonal β-lactam	Tazobactam/ Piperacillin	++	++	++	−
	Aztreonam	−	++	++	−
	Meropenem	++	++	++	++
Polymixin	colistimethate sodium	−	++	++	−
Aminoglycoside	Tobramycin	+	++	++	−
	Amikacin	++	++	++	−

SA, *Staphylococcus aureus* (not MRSA); HI, *Haemophilus influenza*; Pa, *Pseudomonas aeruginosa*; BCC, *Burkholderia cepacia* complex

++ usually good antibiotic cover, + some activity against the organism, - no useful antibacterial activity.

This is intended only as a general guide and should be checked against local and individual antibiotic sensitivities.

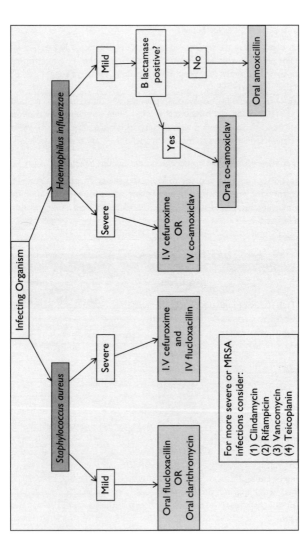

Figure 5.1 Treatment of non-Pseudomonas exacerbations.

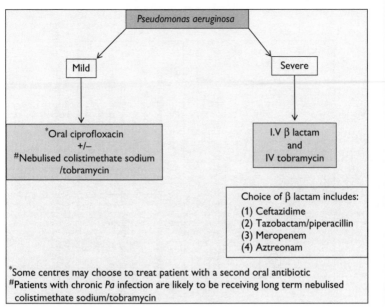

Figure 5.2 Treatment exacerbations in patients with chronic *Pseudomonas aeruginosa* infections.

Exacerbation in patient with chronic Burkholderia cepacia *complex infection*

BCC exhibits high levels of antibiotic resistance including an inherent resistance to colistimethate sodium (see Chapter 3). A combination of 3 intravenous antibiotics should be used for severe exacerbations. The choice of antibiotic should be guided by *in-vitro* sensitivities and the response to previous treatment. A suggested approach is shown in Figure 5.3.

5.4 **IV access devices**

5.4.1 **Long lines**

Long lines are inserted into a large peripheral vein, usually in the antecubital fossa. The catheter is long enough to access the larger, more proximal veins. They are usually left in for the duration of treatment, and can remain in place for up to 4 weeks, unlike small peripheral cannulae which typically require re-insertion every few days. They should be considered in those starting IV antibiotics who do not possess a TIVAD (see later this chapter). They should be flushed with heparinized saline after use.

PICC lines (peripherally inserted central catheters) are similar, although they are usually longer in order to access central veins. PICC line insertion requires special training and radiological confirmation of position.

5.4.2 **Totally implantable/indwelling vascular access device (TIVAD)**

TIVADs, or 'ports', facilitate long-term IV access, avoiding repeated peripheral venous cannula insertion and the irritant effect of infusions on small peripheral veins. A TIVAD consists of a silicone membrane, mounted in a titanium chamber, and inserted subcutaneously

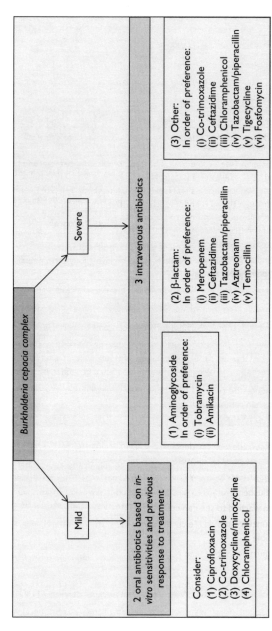

Figure 5.3 Treatment of exacerbations in patients with chronic *Burkholderia cepacia* complex infection. For oral treatments select 1 from each of the 3 boxes, starting with the first listed antibiotic and moving to the next in the list if the selected treatment is unsuitable or has already been selected.

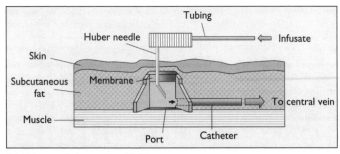

Figure 5.4 Huber needle inserted into TIVAD.

on the chest wall or arm (see Figure 5.4). The chamber is connected to a catheter tunnelled into a central vein. The device is usually inserted by a vascular surgeon under local or general anaesthetic. Venous access is achieved via a Huber (or 'gripper') needle inserted into the chamber through the skin and underlying silicone membrane. The Huber needle remains in place throughout the course of treatment, allowing repeated administration of IV therapies, whilst permitting almost unlimited physical activity.

TIVADS are generally well received by patients, but complications can develop and the mean survival of an individual port is around 3–5 years. Complications occur in around 40%, most commonly catheter occlusion (20% of all TIVADs). Other complications include infection (9%), vascular thrombosis (5%), and catheter displacement (3%) or dis-insertion (2%). TIVAD line infection most commonly presents with symptoms of bacteraemia that may worsen when the TIVAD is used. Confirmed infection is treated by intravenous antibiotics administered via an alternative intravenous line. Surgical removal of the TIVAD is required in 80% of cases. As thrombus may form, there is a risk of septic pulmonary emboli if the infected TIVAD is used. Blood sampling via the TIVAD is convenient for patients, but increases risk of thrombosis (relative risk 2.2). Occlusion or thrombosis can be diagnosed by injecting contrast dye during X-ray screening (a 'linogram'). Incomplete thrombotic occlusion can sometimes be relieved by a fibrinolytic (e.g. Alteplase® 2 mg in 2 ml, left in line for 2 hours and then removed).

Recommendations

- TIVAD should be considered in patients requiring IV antibiotics on a regular basis (i.e. more than 3 times per year), or those with difficult IV access
- TIVADS should only be accessed by appropriately trained healthcare professionals
- Devices must be flushed every 4–6 weeks with heparin solution (5 ml of 100 iu/ml)
- Patients should be warned to seek advice if their TIVAD becomes slow to flush
- If possible, venepuncture should ideally be from a separate, peripheral, vein. In children, this is rarely possible
- Antibiotic levels must never be taken from a TIVAD

5.5 **Non-antibiotic treatments**

5.5.1 **Physiotherapy**

Physiotherapy is used to assist expectoration during an exacerbation. It is widely applied, and has been shown to improve sputum clearance, although there are no controlled clinical trials on its long-term benefits. No specific method of airway clearance has been shown to be superior to any other (see Chapter 4), and the choice is one of patient and physiotherapist preference.

Patients should be assessed on the day of admission and an individualized treatment plan developed and commenced. This should include consideration of airway clearance techniques, inhalation therapy (including oxygen therapy and non-invasive ventilation), and exercise. The treatment plan should be implemented by a physiotherapist who has been trained in CF care. Outcome measures should be used to inform the initial assessment and to monitor the progress throughout the admission. Suitable measures include arterial or capillary blood gases, lung function, sputum weight/volume, sputum consistency, and exercise tolerance. Additional measures such as oxygen saturation, transcutaneous CO_2, spirometry, heart rate, respiratory rate, and symptom scores should be used to monitor the effects of physiotherapy interventions. Preparation for discharge provides a useful platform to review all the components of a physiotherapy maintenance treatment regimen and to ensure treatment burden is managed.

Recommendations

- All patients with an exacerbation should be reviewed early on by a specialist respiratory physiotherapist, and airway clearance assessed. This includes patients considered for HIVAT
- Patients may need additional input or devices to assist expectoration when unwell

- Outcome measures appropriate for the individual patient should be used to assess the success of physiotherapy
- Admission affords a good opportunity to educate and reinforce physiotherapy regimen, and should be provided at least twice per day

5.5.2 **Nutrition**

CF patients will often lose weight during an exacerbation, both because of the increased energy demands of the inflammatory response, and because of reduced appetite. Weight loss or failure to gain weight is an important signs of an exacerbation, particularly in children. Nutritional interventions tailored to the patients' needs may need to be started. These include additional meals and snacks, nutritional supplements, and the introduction of nasogastric or gastrostomy feeding.

Recommendations

- Patients should be weighed before, during, and after treatment
- Patients admitted for an exacerbation should have an early review by a specialist dietitian
- Tailored nutritional interventions should be started in patients with poor nutrition or anorexia

5.5.3 **Management of diabetes**

Abnormal glycaemic control is often more apparent during times of systemic illness, and this can result in protein catabolism and weight loss. It is therefore important to undertake blood glucose monitoring, especially if there is a previous history of impaired glucose handling. In patients with CFRD, insulin requirements usually rise, even if intake is reduced. Patients with impaired glucose tolerance (IGT) who do not normally require insulin may decompensate when unwell, and require the introduction of insulin. Even patients with normal glucose tolerance may have significantly elevated blood glucose (BG) when unwell.

If blood glucose measurements are persistently elevated, insulin should be started or increased.

Recommendations

- A random blood glucose (BG) should be measured in all patients on admission
- A 24-hour glucose profile (i.e. BG before and after meals and 1–2 times overnight) should be considered in all adults and adolescents
- In younger children, random BG should be checked every time bloods are taken for other assays
- BG monitoring should continue throughout the exacerbation if the patient is known to have CFRD, IGT, or if any of the initial BG results were >6 mmol/L
- Patients on enteral feeds should have BG measurements taken before, during, and after at least 1 feed
- Consider starting insulin if BG persistently elevated at any time of day

5.5.4 **Hydration**

Many patients if unwell will not be able to keep up adequate fluid intake, especially if pyrexial, leading to dehydration and salt depletion. This puts them at risk of bowel obstruction, but also leads to dehydrated secretions that are thicker and harder to expel. An important component of treatment for unwell CF patients is therefore IV hydration with 0.9% saline to ensure they are adequately rehydrated. Some units have found that IV aminophylline added to IV hydration overnight (e.g. 500 mg for an adult in 1 L 0.9% saline over 8 hrs) has an additional beneficial effect on mobilisation of secretions. This may relate to effects on airway muscle tone, but no trials have yet been done to investigate this. A final aspect of hydration is to ensure that supplemental oxygen is also humidified. Dry oxygen from cylinders or in hospitals will dehydrate airway secretions and may lead to greater difficulties in airway clearance. This can easily be humidified through special devices.

5.5.5 **Bronchodilators**

Many patients with CF exacerbations also have airway hyper-responsiveness, and an improvement in lung function in hospitalized patients has been shown with regular neb-ulized salbutamol. Many patients will already be using nebulized or inhaled bronchodila-tors before physiotherapy, and these should be continued. Patients with known airway hyper-responsiveness or documented wheeze may also benefit from starting these treat-ments during an exacerbation.

5.5.6 **Nebulized saline**

Nebulized hypertonic saline (7%) may be used to aid sputum clearance during an exacer-bation. However, it can also cause bronchospasm and other adverse reactions and should therefore be preceded by an inhaled or nebulized bronchodilator. A more tolerable alter-native may be 3% or 0.9% (normal) saline, nebulized before physiotherapy, to loosen secre-tions. These therapies can be trialled on an individual basis if patients are experiencing difficulties with airway clearance.

5.5.7 **Oral corticosteroids**

Addition of steroids during exacerbation has not been shown to improve clinical or lung function outcomes in a small study, but it is associated with hyperglycaemia. The use of corticosteroids is not recommended.

5.6 Special considerations

5.6.1 Haemoptysis

Haemoptysis is common in patients with CF. It varies from mild to massive and can be fatal. It is a recognized manifestation of pulmonary exacerbations and all patients with haemoptysis >5 ml should be treated with antibiotics. Most episodes of haemoptysis settle spontaneously but treatment with pro-thrombotic agents such as tranexamic acid or bronchial artery embolization may be required (see Chapter 6). There is no consensus about the use of airway clearance therapies in patients with significant haemoptysis; although the airways need to be cleared there is concern that these therapies may impair clot formation. This has to be decided on a patient by patient basis. Long-term nebulized therapy should be continued. Although there is a lack of evidence in this area, some centres choose to stop nebulized mucolytics (hypertonic saline and dornase alfa) as they can potentially increase the risk of further bleeding.

5.6.2 Pregnancy and antibiotics

Lung function can deteriorate during pregnancy (see Chapter 12), and several courses of IV antibiotics may be required.

- Antibiotics generally considered safe in pregnancy include: β-lactams (penicillins, cephalosporins) and oral erythromycin and clindamycin
- Antibiotics that should not be used include ciprofloxacin, chloramphenicol, metronidazole, and IV colistimethate sodium
- Aminoglycosides are probably safe, but levels need close and careful monitoring. Potential for ototoxicity is greatest in the second trimester, and may occur in the foetus independent of signs of toxicity in the mother

References

Balaguer A. Home versus hospital intravenous antibiotics for cystic fibrosis. *Cochrane Database Syst Rev.* 2012;3:CD001917.

Breen L. Elective versus symptomatic intravenous antibiotic therapy for cystic fibrosis. *Cochrane Database Syst Rev* 2008;3:CD002767.

CF Trust. *Management of cystic fibrosis-related diabetes.* London: CF Trust, 2004.

CF Trust. *Antibiotic treatment for cystic fibrosis*, 3rd edn. London, CF Trust, 2005.

Döring G. Treatment of lung infection in patients with cystic fibrosis: Current and future strategies. *J Cyst Fibrosis* 2012;11:461–79.

Ferkol T, Rosenfield M, Milia CE, et al. Cystic fibrosis pulmonary exacerbations. *J Pediatr* 2006;148:259–64.

Fernandes BN. Duration of intravenous antibiotic therapy in people with cystic fibrosis. *Cochrane Database Syst Rev* 2008;3:CD006682.

Flume PA. Cystic fibrosis pulmonary guidelines. Treatment of pulmonary exacerbations. *Am J Respir Crit Care Med* 2009;180:802–8.

Gibson RL. Pathophysiology and management of pulmonary infections in cystic fibrosis. *Am J Respir Crit Care Med* 2003;168:918–51.

Munck A. Follow–up of 452 TIVADs in cystic fibrosis patients. *Eur Respir J* 2004;23:430–4.

Stenbit AE. (2011). Pulmonary exacerbations in cystic fibrosis. *Curr Opin Pulm Med* 2011;17: 442–7.

Tunney MM. Use of culture and molecular analysis to determine the effect of antibiotic treatment on microbial community diversity and abundance during exacerbation in patients with cystic fibrosis. *Thorax* 2011;66:579–84.

Waters V. Combination antimicrobial susceptibility testing for acute exacerbations in chronic infection of Pseudomonas aeruginosa in cystic fibrosis. *Cochrane Database Syst Rev* 2008;3:CD006961.

Chapter 6

Respiratory complications and management of severe CF lung disease

J Alastair Innes

Key points

- Minor haemoptysis is usually a self-limiting complication of CF infections
- Severe haemoptysis may require bronchial artery embolisation
- Pneumothorax aggravates underlying infection. Tube drainage is appropriate and surgery should be avoided where possible
- Acute respiratory failure complicates acute infections in severe CF lung disease. Non-invasive ventilation (NIV) reduces breathlessness and acidosis without compromising airway clearance, and is therefore preferred to intubation
- Chronic respiratory failure develops insidiously in advanced CF. Hypoxia requires home oxygen. NIV helps to palliate breathlessness and buy time for lung transplant
- Terminal care in CF is challenging. Treatment with palliative intent should be started in discussion with patient and family. Thereafter only treatments which contribute to comfort should be continued, but all such treatments should be actively offered

6.1 Haemoptysis

The extensive bronchiectasis typical of CF lung disease is associated with hypertrophy of the bronchial circulation, predisposing to airway bleeding. Most CF patients experience minor haemoptysis at some stage in their life, usually in the presence of an infective exacerbation. Minor haemoptysis is nearly always self-limiting and patients should be reassured and treated in the conventional way for their airway infection.

A minority of patients develop intermittent episodes of brisk or major haemoptysis, which may amount to several hundred millilitres of blood, with an alarming feeling of choking or even suffocating. Episodes may occur with infection or spontaneously without warning. In patients with CF related portal hypertension, haematemesis from varices is an important differential diagnosis to consider.

6.1.1 Treatment of haemoptysis

Patients should be nursed upright or with the affected side dependent if known. High-flow oxygen is administered, intravenous access secured, clotting checked, and blood cross-matched. An ice-cold drink may reduce haemoptysis by reducing bronchial blood

Box 6.1 Acute management of severe haemoptysis

- Ensure IV access and basic resuscitation (IV fluids to maintain blood pressure, high-flow oxygen to maintain SpO_2)
- Send urgent cross-match, full blood count, and clotting
- Lie patient on side of bleed (if known)
- Provide ice-cold drink if possible
- 1 g tranexamic acid intravenously over 15–20 minutes
- 10 mg vitamin K intravenously
- In severe uncontrolled haemorrhage, patient will need to be intubated. Replace blood loss (either group specific or ORh-ve blood if not previously cross-matched)
- Fresh frozen plasma or cryoprecipitates to correct clotting abnormalities (e.g. in CF liver disease, or if patient given repeated blood transfusions)
- Consider 2 mg terlipressin IV as a stat dose

flow. Chest X-ray may reveal a new infiltrate indicating which lung is bleeding, and a CT scan may reveal abnormally enlarged bronchial arteries, and is usually required before therapeutic embolisation is attempted.

Acute treatment (see Box 6.1) involves resuscitation, and correction of any clotting abnormality using IV vitamin K, fresh frozen plasma, or cryoprecipitate as appropriate. The anti-fibrinolytic agent tranexamic acid can be given as a stat dose intravenously (1 g) and can also be prescribed regularly in those with persistent haemoptysis (1 g QDS orally or intravenously). Terlipressin is a vasopressin analogue licensed for the management of bleeding due to oesophageal varices. Although supporting evidence is limited, this has also been used to control haemoptysis. It is usually given as an IV stat dose of 2 mg, but can be repeated if necessary (1–2 mg every 4–6 hours).

The patient is likely to be anxious and panicked, particularly if this is a new complication or the bleed is large. Consider light sedation to reduce anxiety.

Bronchoscopy in the acute phase is usually both difficult and unhelpful due to the large volume of blood present throughout the bronchial tree, and the coughing it causes. If bleeding persists despite correcting any clotting problem, patients should proceed urgently to bronchial arteriography (see Figure 6.1) and therapeutic bronchial embolization.

In the hands of an experienced interventional radiologist, this procedure is often effective in stopping bleeding. It is common to find that large parts of the bronchial circulation in both lungs are abnormally dilated, and it is usually not possible to identify the bleeding point at angiography. Embolization of all affected dilated vessels may be attempted, although this can be difficult because of multiple vessel origins (intercostals, internal mammary, and aorta). The procedure is intricate and time-consuming, and frequently it is necessary to operate more than once before satisfactory occlusion of all abnormal vessels is achieved. Great care must be taken to avoid obstruction of the anterior spinal artery, which often has a common origin with a bronchial artery, to prevent potentially serious neurological complications.

6.2 **Pneumothorax**

The combination of extensive infective damage to the lung and the increased mechanical stresses due to airflow obstruction predispose CF patients to pneumothorax (Figure 6.2).

Although uncommon, pneumothorax in CF can cause serious additional impairment of respiratory function and may precipitate respiratory failure or occasionally empyema. Pneumothorax should always be considered in patients presenting with acute deterioration

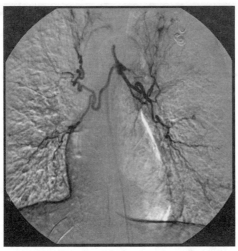

Figure 6.1 Bronchial arteriogram in a patient with CF and massive haemoptysis showing bilateral dilatation and tortuosity of the bronchial arteries.

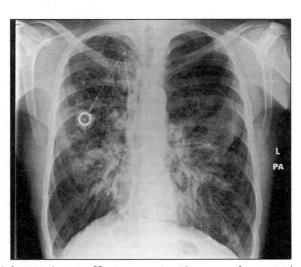

Figure 6.2 Left pneumothorax in a CF patient presenting with symptoms of acute exacerbation.

in their breathing. It is easy to miss, as chest radiology is not always performed for exacerbation of CF lung disease. Radiology to exclude pneumothorax is especially indicated for symptoms of rapid onset, if pleuritic pain is present, or if the breath sounds are clearly asymmetrical in volume.

Pneumothorax may occur as part of an infective exacerbation; if not, then the lung collapse itself usually rapidly precipitates an infective exacerbation, by impairing clearance of sputum. Either way, the patient should receive appropriate antibiotics together with prompt intercostal tube drainage for the pneumothorax.

Persistent air leak is a major problem for some CF patients with pneumothorax, as their underlying condition markedly increases the risks of surgical treatment. Every effort should be made to avoid surgery and to achieve lung re-inflation by simple tube drainage, even if prolonged.

Clinicians are often concerned that pleurodesis procedures performed to treat pneumothorax may compromise patients' future chances of lung transplant surgery. In practice, surgeons generally advise that the priority should always be efficient and rapid resolution of the pneumothorax including pleurodesis or apical pleural abrasion if necessary. Pleurectomy should, however, be avoided to preserve the potential for later transplantation.

6.3 Acute respiratory failure in CF exacerbations

In patients with severe CF lung disease, acute respiratory acidosis can complicate infective exacerbations. Conventional intubation and ventilation with sedation and paralysis in this setting removes all possibility of spontaneous sputum clearance and can therefore lead to progressive airway compromise, with atelectasis, sepsis, and lung collapse. Treatment of acute respiratory failure in CF has been transformed in recent years by the widespread use of non-invasive ventilation (NIV). Not only does this allow patients to continue to participate actively in sputum clearance, it also supports and unloads the respiratory muscles, augmenting minute ventilation and improving gas exchange. Provided the patient is able to tolerate the mask and successfully trigger the ventilator, the result is usually rapid and substantial relief of breathlessness, with gradual resolution of the respiratory acidosis. An additional advantage of NIV is that the conscious patient is able to take short breaks from treatment to expectorate, or to eat and drink.

As CF lung disease advances, it is good practice to discuss in advance with patients the possible future need for NIV and to demonstrate the technique to them before it is needed for a respiratory crisis. This greatly increases the chance of successful NIV when it is needed for acute respiratory failure. Allowing patients to hold the mask to their face and to feel the assisted inspiration increases confidence in what otherwise risks being a frightening and claustrophobic initial experience.

6.3.1 Starting NIV

Initiation of NIV in respiratory exacerbations is appropriate when arterial blood gases indicate acute respiratory failure (consider when arterial H^+ >50 with raised arterial pCO_2). Because lung compliance is reduced in CF, relatively high inspiratory pressures are required to assist lung inflation. A reasonable *starting* point when introducing NIV in CF is 14 cm H_2O inspiratory pressure (IPAP) and 4 cm H_2O expiratory pressure (EPAP); lower inspiratory pressures are often ineffective and the patient may feel the equipment is encumbering rather than assisting breathing. Serial arterial blood gases should show reducing H^+ and pCO_2 levels. Patients who do not respond may require increased IPAP, but gastric distension with air may become a limiting factor as IPAP increases above 20 cm H_2O.

Success and symptomatic relief are greatest when patients have high respiratory drive but are too tired or have such severe airway obstruction that they cannot achieve sufficient minute ventilation unassisted. Drowsy patients respond much less well to NIV, and sedation should be avoided or used with great caution in this situation. In all cases, care should be taken to ensure a good mask fit with minimal leak.

6.4 Chronic respiratory failure in CF

6.4.1 **Chronic type I respiratory failure**

In moderate CF lung disease, hypoxia is the main gas exchange abnormality (type 1 respiratory failure) due to the passage of blood through unventilated or poorly ventilated lung units. Hypoxia is exacerbated overnight when minute ventilation declines physiologically, and overnight monitoring of oxygen saturation is helpful to detect this problem. Oxygen concentrators fitted in the patient's home permit long-term oxygen therapy, which is usually only required overnight in the initial stages. Patients with exertional symptoms may be desaturating during exercise even if resting blood gases are satisfactory. Oximetry during treadmill walking can detect this problem, and exercise tolerance and breathlessness scores should be compared with and without supplementary oxygen. Ambulatory oxygen can be provided using conventional portable cylinders or cylinders which can be filled at home from special 'Homefill' oxygen concentrators. Oxygen conserving devices which release oxygen only during inspiration significantly increase the duration of therapy available from lightweight portable cylinders. Liquid oxygen is an alternative method of supply for home and portable oxygen therapy but is not universally available.

6.4.2 **Chronic type II respiratory failure**

As disease progresses, type II respiratory failure with CO_2 retention eventually supervenes as the number of normally functioning lung units declines, and ventilation/perfusion mismatch becomes more generalized. Patients may notice morning headache, a symptom which should trigger measurement of morning arterial blood gases. For those with chronic elevation of arterial pCO_2, home NIV is a useful option for supporting the patient pending a lung transplant, and can buy sufficient time for transplant to occur. Treatment is normally initiated in hospital, and in the early stages patients may benefit by using it only overnight at home.

The place of chronic non-invasive ventilation in the palliative treatment of end-stage CF lung disease in patients who are not listed for lung transplantation is more contentious. A careful clinical assessment of the individual patient's needs should be made and a frank discussion of the options with the patient and their family is always required. Some patients with high respiratory drive who are distressed by chronic breathlessness may find NIV helpful in the palliation of breathlessness; however, other patients feel distressed and claustrophobic when presented with NIV apparatus, and prefer a pharmacological approach to the management of breathlessness.

6.5 Terminal care for advanced CF lung disease

Managing death with dignity in a young patient is extremely challenging for the whole multidisciplinary team. A key challenge in many cases is identifying the point at which the hope of a lung transplant rescuing the patient from respiratory failure is replaced by the need to change tack and palliate symptoms, recognizing that death is inevitable and imminent. Patients and families differ in the extent to which they welcome discussion of these issues, but team members must offer the opportunity for such discussions if they are wanted.

The clinical situation is usually that of a prolonged infective exacerbation which has failed to respond to appropriate antibiotics. The patient may be febrile, breathless, and also frightened. They are often sleep-deprived and also undernourished as appetite is inevitably poor at such times.

Ideally, the decision to manage with predominantly palliative intent should be a positive one following an open discussion among the team, patient, and family. It should be stressed that treatment is not being withdrawn or withheld; rather, it is being refocused on symptom control. Each of the patient's treatments should be re-evaluated using the question 'is this helping the patient's comfort?' Although antibiotics may not be reversing the progress of the patient's disease, they may be limiting sepsis and fever, and are often continued for symptomatic benefit. Oxygen is useful palliation for breathlessness in hypoxic patients, and should be humidified if the concentration used is over 28%. Intravenous fluids should be given to prevent uncomfortable dehydration. Beyond this, any pain should be addressed with appropriate analgesia, then the focus should move to the optimal control of breathlessness, which is usually the most frightening symptom.

Morphine given orally or subcutaneously is very effective palliation for breathlessness and the dose should be titrated upwards according to response. In very anxious or panicky patients, benzodiazepines may be added to alleviate distress. The goal of treatment is to avoid at all costs the situation where the dying patient is 'fighting for breath'. Careful empathetic nursing supervision and constant dose monitoring and adjustment are necessary to avoid this. Morphine syringe pumps are a useful option in some patients.

The best outcome is a peaceful sedated state where the patient is still able to communicate freely with their family between periods of rest and sleep.

Bereavement support for the family is an important part of holistic CF care and should not be overlooked.

References

Efrati O, Modan-Moses D, Barak A, et al. Long-term non-invasive positive pressure ventilation among cystic fibrosis patients awaiting lung transplantation. *Isr Med Assoc J* 2004;6:527–30.

Flume PA. Mogayzel PJ Jr. Robinson KA. et al. Cystic fibrosis pulmonary guidelines: pulmonary complications: hemoptysis and pneumothorax. *Am J Resp Crit Care Med* 2010;182(3):298–306.

MacDuff A, Tweedie J, McIntosh L, et al. Pneumothorax in cystic fibrosis: prevalence and outcomes in Scotland. *J Cyst Fibrosis* 2010;Jul;9(4):246–9.

Sands D, Repetto T, Dupont LJ, et al. End of life care for patients with cystic fibrosis. *J Cyst Fibrosis* 2011;10 Suppl 2:S37–44.

Chapter 7

Gastrointestinal disease and nutrition

Christopher Taylor and Sally Connolly

Key points

- Lung function and survival correlate with nutritional status
- 85% are pancreatic insufficient, requiring enzyme supplementation
- Pancreatic enzyme replacement dosage should not exceed 10 000 lipase units/kg body weight or 1000 U/4 g dietary fat
- Gastro-oesophageal reflux is common and may present with increasing respiratory disease
- Around 10% develop liver cirrhosis, treated initially with ursodeoxycholic acid
- Poor weight gain should prompt a dietary review. Calorie/protein supplementation may be required with NG or PEG feeding

7.1 Introduction

Although progressive respiratory failure is the major cause of death, CF is a multi-system disease with important consequences for the liver and bowel. Gastrointestinal disease is the earliest clinical manifestation of CF, and may present antenatally with hyper-echoic or dilated fetal bowel on sonography. The first clear detailed clinical and pathological description of CF, in 1938, was of 49 patients with neonatal intestinal obstruction, intestinal and respiratory complications. CF was originally considered as part of the 'coeliac syndrome', since both may present with malabsorption (Figure 7.1). Prior to the development of the sweat test and intestinal biopsy, establishing a diagnosis on clinical grounds was far from easy.

The development of effective pancreatic extracts, and the demonstration by the Toronto clinic in the 1970s that aggressive management of nutritional failure improved survival, was a significant advance. These days, the importance of good nutrition and optimization of BMI are well recognized, although respiratory complications have eclipsed gastrointestinal complications as the primary cause of mortality. Underweight patients have poorer clinical outcomes, and low weight (weight for height <85%, or BMI <17 in adults) is associated with increased post-transplant mortality.

Gastrointestinal involvement in cystic fibrosis extends from mouth to anus. In addition to the gastrointestinal complications described in this chapter, dental enamel mineral abnormalities are also more common in CF children.

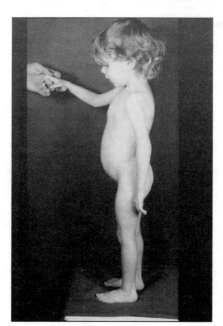

Figure 7.1 CF presenting as malabsorption.

7.2 **Intestinal disease and obstruction**

7.2.1 **Physiology**

The cells (enterocytes) which line the intestinal tract have a primary role in the absorption of nutrients, electrolytes, and water. Enterocytes, however, also secrete electrolytes and water into the gut lumen. This secretion maintains the fluidity of the intestinal contents and provides Na^+ for Na^+-dependent nutrient absorption. The secretory process involves Cl^- secretion via apical cystic fibrosis transmembrane conductance regulator (CFTR) channels, coupled with an inhibition of Na^+ and water movement into the cell. Anion movement into the gut causes Na^+ to move into the lumen via the paracellular pathway, with water following osmotically.

In the CF intestine there is a failure of CFTR-mediated Cl^- secretion, coupled with enhanced Na^+ and Na^+-linked nutrient absorption, leading to excessive dehydration of the luminal contents. This contributes to the development of the intestinal symptoms experienced by CF patients.

7.2.2 **Meconium ileus**

Meconium ileus (MI) is the earliest clinical manifestation of CF, affecting 10–20% of CF infants (see also Chapter 2). Overall survival is currently over 90%.

Presentation

The condition presents within the first day or two of life with signs of intestinal obstruction (Figure 7.2):

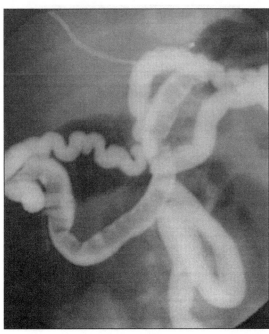

Figure 7.2 Contrast enema from infant with meconium ileus. There is a microcolon with radiolucent areas in the terminal ileum where contrast has mixed with pellets of meconium.

- abdominal distension (96%)
- bilious vomiting (49%)
- delayed passage of meconium (36%)

MI can be divided into complicated (39–46%) and simple forms, the former depending upon the presence of associated volvulus, atresias, perforation, peritonitis, and/or pseudocyst formation. Survival in complex MI is 67%, compared with 93% in uncomplicated disease. Long-term follow-up suggests that survivors show similar hepato-biliary, nutritional, functional, and respiratory status to non-MI CF. Despite the strong association with pancreatic exocrine insufficiency, MI is also seen in the absence of CF and occurs in pancreatic-sufficient individuals with CF.

Investigations

Plain abdominal X-ray typically shows dilated intestinal loops and may also show a 'ground glass' appearance, representing small air bubbles mixed with meconium. Contrast enema may show microcolon with obstruction in the terminal ileum, as in Figure 7.2.

Management

In uncomplicated cases, barium enema plus N-acetylcysteine, combined with IV rehydration, may be sufficient to relieve obstruction. Perforation, volvulus, atresia, or failed medical therapy require laporotomy.

7.2.3 **Gastro-oesophageal reflux disease (GORD)**

Incidence

An increased prevalence of gastro-oesophageal reflux has been reported in infants, children and adults with CF. Based on a fractional reflux time >10% with an oesophageal pH <4.0, almost 20% of CF infants <6 months of age will have GORD. However, the normal range for the reflux index during the first 12 months of life encompasses about 10% of infants (95th percentile), decreasing from 13% at birth to 8% at 12 months. Incidence figures for reflux in older children with CF vary between 25% and 100%, depending on patient selection. Similar high rates have been reported in CF adolescents and adults with suggestive symptomatology.

Effect on lungs

GORD may adversely affect lung disease by aspiration and reflex bronchospasm. Impedance-pH monitoring combined with bronchoalveolar lavage for bile acids has shown that both acid (pH <4) and weakly acid (pH 4–7) reflux are common in CF even in the absence of typical reflux symptoms. Oesophageal manometry has also demonstrated that GORD is not only secondary to cough, but that cough also follows reflux episodes.

Medical management

Symptomatic reflux, or in patients in whom there is a clinical suspicion in the absence of definite symptoms, require proton pump inhibitors (e.g. omeprazole 2 mg/Kg/day—dose should be split if on overnight feeds). Motility agents can also be used (e.g. domperidone 200–400 ug/kg qid pre feeds).

Fundoplication

The outcome following fundoplication in children with CF is similar to that reported in large series in children without CF. Boesch and colleagues (2007) reported high rate of recurrent GORD (48%) and little apparent benefit for either nutritional or pulmonary outcomes, although children with an FEV_1 of less than 60% predicted at the time of fundoplication exhibited an improvement in FEV_1 decline post intervention. A more recent study in a larger cohort of adults and children with CF, however, found fundoplicated subjects required fewer courses of intravenous antibiotics in the first year after surgery compared with the year before and had improved weight gain and a slower decline in FEV_1.

7.2.4 **Distal ileal obstruction syndrome (DIOS)**

Presentation

DIOS, previously known as meconium ileus equivalent, occurs predominantly in patients over 15 years of age and presents either acutely, with signs of abdominal obstruction, or more commonly sub-acutely, with cramping abdominal pain and relative constipation.

Conditions that lead to dehydration may precipitate DIOS and should be avoided.

Diagnosis

The diagnosis is usually made on clinical grounds and can be confirmed with a plain abdominal film if there is clinical doubt: this characteristically shows a speckled faecal gas pattern in the right lower quadrant whereas constipation will show faecal accumulation throughout the bowel. Clinical examination may reveal a (tender) mass in the right iliac fossa. Volvulus may rarely occur.

Differential diagnosis

- Appendicitis
- Appendix abscess
- Mucocoele of the appendix
- Constipation
- Intussusception
- Fibrosing colonopathy
- Crohn's disease

Treatment

- Optimize pancreatic enzyme supplementation to control steatorrhoea
- Avoid dehydration and drugs that may inhibit gut motility
- Mucolytics—N-acetylcysteine (10–20 g in 100 ml water), though this treatment is now little used
- Gastrografin®—(diatrizoate) orally or rectally (oral, <7 years, 50 ml; >7 years 100 ml: dose can be repeated after 4 hours if there is no response). Patients should take at least as much water by mouth as the volume of Gastrografin®. (Alternative preparations including Citramag® and Klean-Prep® may also be used)
- Intravenous rehydration. Patients are typically dehydrated and can sequester considerable fluid volumes in obstructed bowels

7.2.5 **Diseases of the appendix**

Appendiceal disease is often misdiagnosed as DIOS and should be considered in any patient with a right lower quadrant mass. Complications, including perforation and abscess formation, are increased, reflecting delay in diagnosis.

In CF, the appendix is frequently abnormal on ultrasound with scans showing either mucoid appendix (16%), or a pathologically thickened appendiceal wall.

7.2.6 **Constipation**

Constipation is common in CF at all ages: more than 70% of CF patients over 30 years of age have signs and symptoms of constipation. Small bowel and colonic transit is prolonged; studies suggest a mouth to anus transit of between 25 and 55 hours, versus a normal range of 12–48 hours.

7.2.7 **Rectal prolapse**

Protrusion of the rectal mucous membrane through the anus is commonly seen in association with diarrhoeal diseases and constipation. It should always be considered as a presenting sign of CF (10–13%). Rectal prolapse is rare after 4 years of age.

7.2.8 **Fibrosing colonopathy**

Fibrosing colonopathy is a rare condition seen almost exclusively in children with CF. It chiefly affects the caecum and ascending colon. Fibrosing colonopathy is characterized by submucosal fibrosis, with thickening of the muscularis propria leading to stricture formation. The disorder is associated with the use of high-dose pancreatic enzyme supplementation (>10 000 U lipase/kg/day). Evidence that the methacrylic acid copolymer enteric coating of some enzymes preparations predisposed to colonopathy needs confirmation.

7.2.9 **Pancreatitis**

All patients with CF have abnormal pancreatic function; however, patients with mild disease (15–20%) may have sufficient pancreatic enzyme production to prevent overt steatorrhoea and promote normal weight gain. Pancreatic-sufficient patients are more susceptible to episodes of pancreatitis, which can lead to progressive loss of pancreatic function and eventual pancreatic insufficiency. Acute pancreatitis is managed as per non-CF-related pancreatitis with fluids, analgesia, and resting the gut. Most episodes settle spontaneously.

Patients with recurrent episodes of acute pancreatitis may benefit from introduction of low-dose pancreatic enzyme supplements to inhibit pancreatic secretion and thereby reduce the frequency of attacks.

7.2.10 **Malignancy**

Whilst there is no overall increased risk of cancer, CF patients have a significantly increased predisposition to digestive tract malignancy—around 6.5 times that of age-matched non-CF population.

Tumours have been identified in the oesophagus, stomach, small and large intestine, and biliary tract. Pancreatic cancer may also be found in association with cystic fibrosis, although the risk appears to relate to inherited pancreatic cancers, which represent approximately 5–10% of all pancreatic cancers.

7.2.11 **CF and other enteropathies**

Although steatorrhoea and azotorrhoea (excessive loss of proteins in stool) principally reflect pancreatic exocrine failure, absorption may also be compromised by associated intolerances and enteropathies. Coeliac disease has been reported in association with CF, as have other enteropathies including cow's milk protein intolerance, lactose intolerance, and Crohn's disease. These alternative diagnoses should be considered in CF patients not responding to appropriate CF nutritional support (see later this chapter).

7.2.12 **Eosinophilic oesoapagitis**

Eosinophilic oesophagitis, a TH-2-driven allergen-mediated disease presenting with dysphagia, or reflux-like symptoms, has recently been described in a small cohort of patients with CF. Diagnosis is by demonstrating >15 eosinophils/HPF in oesophageal tissue and treatment is by exclusion diet +/− immunosupressives.

7.3 **Nutrition**

7.3.1 **Pathophysiology of malabsorption**

The pancreas is part of a complex digestive system including liver, gallbladder, and intestinal secretions. Digestive enzymes are produced in the glandular cells (acini), stored in secretory vesicles (zymogens), and released into the proximal duodenum mixed with large volumes of bicarbonate-rich fluid secreted by the pancreatic duct cells. Each day, 6–20 g of digestive enzymes are secreted into the duodenum in 2.5 L of bicarbonate-rich fluid.

Enzyme secretion occurs in response to food in the proximal duodenum and is regulated by hormonal and neural interactions, involving regulatory peptides and neurotransmitters from the gut, the pancreas, and the vagus nerve including secretin, CCK, neurotensin, motilin, and PYY. Proteolytic enzymes are secreted as pro-enzymes which are activated by enterokinases.

In CF, pancreatic secretions are reduced, with low volumes of fluid and bicarbonate. This causes duct obstruction, and retention and activation of secreted pro-enzymes in the pancreatic ducts, resulting in destruction and fibrosis of the pancreas itself. This process begins *in utero* and continues after birth leading to functional exocrine pancreatic insufficiency (PI) in the majority of CF infants. Mild mutations in the CFTR gene such as R117H and A455E, however, are associated with sufficient pancreatic function to prevent overt steatorrhoea (fatty stool; frequently floating, foul smelling, and pale coloured due to the presence of undigested lipid), but may have a degree of malabsorption particularly of fat-soluble vitamins.

Enzymes are activated on reaching the intestine but require an optimum pH >5.5. The pH in the proximal intestine is usually between 5.5 and 6.5, but failure of pancreatic bicarbonate production in CF means that stomach acid entering the duodenum is inadequately neutralized. The pH in the CF duodenum is therefore often much lower than 5.0, inhibiting enzyme activity. If the pH falls further (to less than 4.0) any enzyme, either produced by the pancreas or taken in the form of pancreatic enzyme-replacment therapy, will be degraded and food will not be digested.

Fecal elastase is a reliable marker of exocrine PI and can be used to monitor pancreatic function over time.

Approximately 60% of CF newborns are already pancreatic-insufficient, and the majority of the remaining CF infants will become pancreatic-insufficient by the end of their first year. Malabsorption is, however, not simply the result of defective enzyme secretion alone but results from 5 separate but interdependent processes:

- Pancreatic insufficiency
- Inactivation of enzymes by pepsin and hyperacidity in upper intestine
- Failure of CFTR-mediated intestinal HCO_3^- secretion
- Deranged bile acid function
- Defective fat absorption

7.3.2 **Bile acid dysfunction**

In the intestine, bile acids are secreted into the lumen of the duodenum where they contribute to the processing of dietary fat. They also activate secretory processes in the intestine. Bile acids are conserved by active reabsorption via a Na^+-dependent mechanism localized to the enterocytes in the terminal ileum. From here, they enter the portal circulation and are returned to the liver for re-secretion into the bile. This enterohepatic circulation of bile acids is extremely efficient, with less than 10% escaping reabsorption and being lost in the feces each day.

The first step in the uptake of bile acids involves a Na^+ gradient-driven co-transporter, the ileal bile acid transporter (IBAT), located on the luminal membranes of ileal enterocytes. This operates in a similar fashion to the co-transporters responsible for Na^+-linked nutrient absorption, whose activities are altered in CF.

Thus, two aspects of bile acid function in the intestine, their stimulation of secretion and their active reuptake by the terminal ileum, may be affected by CF. Bile acid malabsorption is a constant finding in untreated CF. Bile acids are also bound to the undigested protein fraction of the stool, making them unavailable for reabsorption. Fecal losses of bile acids range from 24–57 mg/kg/day. This leads to depletion of the bile acid pool and impaired fat absorption.

7.3.3 **Pancreatic enzyme replacement therapy (PERT)**

Pancreatic enzymes have been available since the 1930s. Early preparations were from pig pancreas, prepared by alcohol extraction. They contained the three major enzyme groups, amylase, lipase, and trypsin, but with considerable batch-to-batch variation in enzyme activity. Nevertheless, they increased fat absorption from 50–60% to 75%, improved growth, and normalized blood and tissue concentrations of fat-soluble vitamins. Much activity was, however, lost through the action of gastric acid and pepsin as the powders passed through the stomach. This led to the introduction of enteric-coated tablets in the 1980s. They were designed to dissolve in the duodenum at pH >5. Unfortunately, many tablets were retained in the stomach, and for those that reached the duodenum, the pH was often too low to promote enzyme activity.

In 1988, Meyer and colleagues showed that 1.4 mm spheres moved from the stomach at the same rate as a test meal and from this work most of our current PERT has evolved. These enteric-coated microspheres and mini-tablets have further improved fat absorption to 85–90%.

High-strength enzymes, containing 22–25 000 units lipase/capsule were introduced in the early 1990s. These preparations gave equal or better control of malabsorption with a significant reduction in capsule consumption but as individual dosages increased, clusters of patients with strictures in the large bowel began to be reported. Fibrosing colonopathy, as it was later called, has been shown to be related to high enzyme intakes. Better control of enzyme dosage and changes in enzyme formulation has reduced new cases of fibrosing colonopathy to very low levels.

7.3.4 **PERT dosage**

PERT is readily available in the form of enteric-coated porcine pancreatic extract in strengths ranging from 3000–40 000 U lipase/capsule. Dose requirements vary but are in the order of 1– 4000 U lipase/gram dietary fat.

Enzyme activity is affected by the following:

- Gastric emptying and gut motility
- Whether taken fasted or after food
- Size/volume of meal
- Composition of meal
  - solid/liquid
  - % and type of fat
- Intestinal pH
- Liver/bile acid function

7.3.5 **Role of the dietitian**

CF is a multi-system disease and best managed by a multidisciplinary team in specialist centres. An experienced specialist dietitian who understands the level of dietetic support required and has expertise in invasive nutritional support is an essential part of the team.

7.4 **Management of poor weight gain**

7.4.1 **Investigations**

Nutritional problems in patients with CF should not be assumed to be secondary to pancreatic insufficiency. Coeliac disease should be excluded by appropriate serologic tests and evidence of lactose intolerance and bacterial overgrowth sought, especially in infants and children who have had surgery for meconium ileus.

Investigation of ongoing malabsorption in CF

- Coeliac screen
  - Tissue transglutaminase or endomyseal antibodies
- Lactose tolerance test
- Breath H_2 test for bacterial overgrowth
- Liver function tests
  - Transaminases
  - Clotting
- Endoscopy and small intestinal biopsy
- Hepatic ultrasound scan
- Contrast meal and follow through
- Abdominal MR

7.4.2 Management

General measures

Nutritional status in CF has been shown to correlate with lung function and survival. Energy requirements are increased to 120–150% of those needed by healthy individuals of the same age and sex. This reflects increased energy demands of the disease and malabsorption of protein and calories, which persists despite PERT therapy. Nevertheless, good nutritional status can be achieved in most individuals by combining a high-calorie, high-protein diet with adequate PERT.

Deficient intake is the chief reason for growth failure in patients with CF lung disease, particularly during exacerbations when lean tissue is rapidly lost. Support with whole protein or juice supplements may help maintain body mass in the short term, but in the long term, oral supplements appear to give no benefits in terms of measures of body composition or lung function.

With advancing lung disease, energy expenditure rises and anorexia is common, leading to energy imbalance. The following steps should be taken before embarking on invasive nutritional support:

- Optimize oral intake
- Review adequacy of PERT
  - If dose >10 000 lipase units/kg body weight add a proton pump inhibitor (see above) to enhance PERT function (may need to be given BD if on overnight feeds)
- Aggressive treatment of lung infection
- Exclude and treat GORD
- Exclude CF-related diabetes mellitus

7.4.3 NG and PEG feeding

Enteral tube feeding should be used if, after oral supplements, weight for height <85% in children or BMI <18.5 kg/m^2 in adults. Other indications include failure to gain weight over a 6-month period (despite oral supplementation), inadequate weight gain in pregnancy, or progressive deterioration in pulmonary status in an underweight patient. Nasogastric (NG) feeding is simple and can be used successfully for short-term support during respiratory exacerbations, as an episodic boost to maintain growth or as a trial prior to gastrostomy feeding. This can be left in place, or re-inserted for each feed, depending on patient preference.

Where longer-term support is required, percutaneous endoscopic gastrostomy (PEG) placement should be considered. Patients with portal gastropathy may be unsuitable for PEG, and percutaneous jejunostomy is an alternative. Feeds are usually given overnight as a complement to normal food. Careful monitoring of blood glucose is necessary when feeds are first introduced, and some previously non-diabetic patients may require insulin supplementation with feeds.

PEG insertion may initially be perceived negatively by patients and must be carefully timed. This is especially important in advanced disease, since post-operative pain can inhibit cough and mucus clearance and exacerbate lung disease. Patients should be reassured that the gastrostromy button, on the upper abdomen, is easily concealed by clothing, and both more discrete and easier to use than NG tubes. Once in situ, many patients find the nutritional support facilitated by the PEG tube relieves the stress and anxiety of daytime meals.

Both polymeric (whole protein) and elemental/semi-elemental feeds can be used to support nutrition. Elemental feeds generally contain a mixture of long- and medium-chain triglycerides, have a higher osmolarity and lower calorie density than polymeric feeds. Polymeric feeds with PERT appear as effective as elemental feeds in promoting weight gain. An enzyme dose based on the main-meal dose is advised with the dose split 50% at the start of the feed and a further 50% given during or immediately after the feed: enzymes should not be put down the tube but where oral dosage is not possible, PERT can be dissolved in bicarbonate and delivered via the tube. It is not considered necessary to wake patients to take enzymes.

7.5 **Hepato-biliary disease**

A variety of biliary tract and hepatic complications have been reported in CF patients. They include gallbladder diseases comprising micro-gallbladder and cholelithiasis, and bile duct abnormalities including sclerosing cholangitits and bile duct strictures. Hepatic complications include steatosis, focal biliary cirrhosis, multi-lobular cirrhosis, neonatal cholestasis, and drug hepatotoxicity. Liver cirrhosis is the single most important cause of non-pulmonary death accounting for 2.5% of CF mortality.

7.5.1 **Incidence**

Almost all cases present in the first 2 decades of life and may reflect the influence of modifier genes, particularly mutations in the α-1-antitrypsin, mannose-binding lectin, and glutathione-S-transferase genes, on CFTR function. Evidence of chronic liver disease is found in 25% of CF patients but less than 10% will progress to cirrhosis. Liver failure (2–3%) and variceal bleeding (1–2%) are rare. Most cases of chronic liver disease are identified by ultrasound scans carried out as part of routine follow-up in patients with an established diagnosis of CF or detection of hepato-splenomegaly on clinical examination.

Evidence of portal hypertension may develop before there is enough liver damage to affect liver synthetic function. Liver function tests may only be mildly abnormal or indeed normal and do not accurately reflect disease severity (see section 7.5.4).

7.5.2 **Pathogenesis**

The characteristic hepatic lesion in CF is focal biliary cirrhosis (Figure 7.3), although fatty infiltration is also seen. In the liver, CFTR is localized to the cholangiocytes in the intra-hepatic bile ducts and gallbladder epithelial cells: defective chloride secretion inhibits the hydration of canalicular-produced bile, leading to plugging of intra-hepatic bile ducts. In addition, intra-hepatic biliary epithelial cells produce excessive mucus, composed of proteoglycans, which further contributes to the viscosity of CF bile. Plugging within the

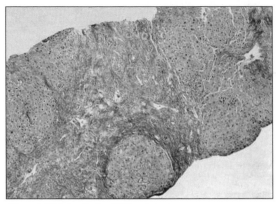

Figure 7.3 Liver biopsy (×100) showing focal biliary cirrhosis.

intra-hepatic bile ducts exposes the hepatocytes to a high concentration of potentially toxic bile acids leading to inflammation and scaring.

Risk factors

- Male gender
- Pancreatic insufficiency
- Severe CFTR mutations
- Meconium ileus

7.5.3 **Treatment**

Optimizing the nutritional status is of prime importance and may require supplemental feeds. Ursodeoxycholic acid is an anti-inflammatory that also stimulates cholangiocellular calcium-dependent secretion of chloride and bicarbonate ions, thus promoting bile flow. It is widely used to treat CF liver disease and has few side effects. It appears to normalize liver function tests, but long-term efficacy remains uncertain. Liver transplantation has been successfully undertaken in the presence of isolated liver decompensation with maintained pulmonary function.

Portal hypertension can lead to the development of oesophageal varices. These are treated as in non-CF patients, with variceal banding or transjugular intra-hepatic portosystemic shunting (TIPPS).

7.5.4 **Monitoring**

The wide variation in the reported prevalence of CF liver disease probably reflects marked under-diagnosis. CF liver disease should be actively sought as part of the annual review. If evidence of liver disease is found, other causes of liver disease such as infection, drug reactions, alpha-1-antityrpsin deficiency and Wilson's disease should be excluded. Liver biopsy may be required for confirmation of diagnosis. Often the only feature of CF-related liver disease is an enlarged liver; splenomegaly if present, is a sign that the liver disease is more advanced and that portal hypertension is also present. Ultrasound should be carried out as part of the annual assessment. It is able to distinguish between normal and abnormal liver texture, the presence of steatosis, fibrosis, cirrhosis, and the presence or absence of splenomegaly. Doppler ultrasound can measure venous and arterial wave forms which provide information on blood flow, dampened or reversed flow indicating more advanced cirrhosis, and portal hypertension. Scoring systems such as the Williams/Westaby score have been devised for CF liver disease, which allow comparison between serial ultrasounds to be made. Other non-invasive methods of testing for liver fibrosis such as transient elastography and acoustic-radiation-force impulse (ARFI) may become useful tools in CF liver disease and enable more accurate monitoring of disease progression.

References

Goralski JL, Lercher DM, Davis SD, et al. Eosinophilic esophagitis in cystic fibrosis: a case series and review of the literature. *J Cyst Fibrosis* 2013 Jan;12(1):9–14.

Ledson MJ, Tran J, Walshaw MJ. Prevalence and mechanisms of gastro-oesophageal reflux in adult cystic fibrosis patients. *J R Soc Med* 1998;91:7–9.

Littlewood JM. Cystic fibrosis: gastrointestinal complications. *Br Med Bull* 1992;48:847–59.

McPartlin JF, Dickson JAS, Swain VA. (1972). Meconium ileus. Immediate and longterm survival. *Arch Dis Child* 1972;47(252):207–10.

Pencharz PB, Durie PR. Pathogenesis of malnutrition in cystic fibrosis, and its treatment. *Clin Nutr* 2000;19:387–94.

Sheikh SI, Ryan-Wenger NA, McCoy KS. Outcomes of surgical management of severe GERD in patients with cystic fibrosis. *Pediatr Pulmonol* 2013 Jun;48(6):556–62.

Smyth RL, Walters S. Oral calorie supplements for cystic fibrosis. *Cochrane Database Syst Rev* 2007;24(1):CD000406.

UK CF Trust Nutrition Working Group. *Nutritional management of cystic fibrosis*. UK CF Trust, April 2002.

Westaby D. Cystic Fibrosis: Liver Disease. In: *Cystic Fibrosis in the 21st Century* (eds Bush A, Alton EWFW, Davies JC, Griesenbach U, Jaffe A), *Prog Respir Res* 2006;34:251–61.

Chapter 8

Cystic fibrosis-related diabetes

Stephen MP O'Riordan and Antoinette Moran

Key points

- Diabetes is the most common comorbidity in CF, with a prevalence of about 50% by 30–50 years of age

- CF-related diabetes (CFRD) is generally insidious in onset, and screening with annual oral glucose-tolerance testing (OGTT) is recommended

- Continuous glucose monitoring (CGM) can detect abnormalities earlier than OGTT. However, the clinical significance of these early changes remains uncertain

- CFRD is predominantly an insulin-insufficiency state, leading to protein catabolism, weight loss, pulmonary function decline, and increased mortality from CF lung disease. Clinical decline can be seen prior to diagnosis of diabetes, in the pre-diabetic, but insulin-insufficient phase of the disease

- Insulin is the only recommended medical therapy for CFRD. Early intervention with insulin has been shown to reverse clinical deterioration, even in those with mild diabetes (i.e. without fasting hyperglycaemia)

- Annual urine albumin screening and retinal exams are recommended for those diagnosed with CFRD with fasting hyperglycaemia for a duration of 5 years or more

---

8.1 Introduction

Cystic fibrosis-related diabetes (CFRD) is the most common comorbidity in persons with CF. While CFRD shares features of both type 1 (T1D) and type 2 diabetes (T2D), there are important differences which necessitate a unique approach to diagnosis and management (see Table 8.1). Factors specific to CF that variably affect glucose metabolism include chronic respiratory infection and inflammation, increased energy expenditure, malnutrition, glucagon deficiency, and gastrointestinal abnormalities (malabsorption, altered gastric emptying, and intestinal motility, CF liver disease). The treatments necessary to treat and prolong life in CF, including their unique dietary requirements, must always be followed as a first priority, with diabetes care adjusted accordingly.

8.2 Definitions

CFRD falls at one end of a spectrum of progressive glucose tolerance abnormalities (see Table 8.2). Few CF patients have completely normal glucose levels at all times. The earliest change is variable, intermittent post-prandial hyperglycaemia which can be picked up by continuous glucose monitoring (CGM) even in subjects with normal glucose tolerance

Table 8.1 Comparison of different forms of diabetes

	Type 1	Type 2	CFRD
Onset	Acute	Insidious	Insidious
Peak age of onset	Children, youth	Adults	18–24 yr
Autoantibody positive?	YES	NO	NO
Insulin secretion	Absent	Decreased	Decreased
Insulin sensitivity	Somewhat decreased	Severely decreased	Somewhat decreased*
Treatment	Insulin	Diet, oral meds, insulin	Insulin
Microvasular complications	YES	YES	YES
Macrovascular complications	YES	YES	NO
Cause of Death	Cardiovascular	Cardiovascular	Pulmonary

*Insulin sensitivity becomes severely decreased during acute illness.

Table 8.2 Abnormal glucose tolerance categories in CF

Category	FPG (mmol/L)	2 hr glucose (mmol/L)	Notes
Normal (NGT)	<7.0	<7.8	All glucose levels <11.1
Indeterminate (INDET)	<7.0	<7.8	Mid-OGTT glucose ≥11.1
Impaired (IGT)	<7.0	7.8–11.1	
CFRD FH-	<7.0	≥11.1	
CFRD FH+	≥7.0		

FPG = fasting plasma glucose; FH = fasting hyperglycemia

(NGT) by OGTT testing. This may be followed by indeterminate glycaemia (mid-OGTT glucose elevation in a subject whose fasting and 2-hour glucose levels are normal), impaired glucose tolerance (IGT), diabetes without fasting hyperglycaemia (CFRD FH-), and diabetes with fasting hyperglycaemia (CFRD FH+). Isolated impaired fasting glucose is sometimes found in CF, but most patients tend to maintain a normal fasting glucose level even when their post-prandial or 2-hour OGTT glucose is in the diabetic range.

8.2.1 **Diagnosis**

The diagnostic criteria for CFRD were updated by the CFRD Guidelines Committee in 2010. The diagnosis of CFRD is determined by the presence of any of:

- Fasting hyperglycaemia
- Random hyperglycaemia in the presence of classic symptoms
- Diabetic pattern on oral glucose tolerance test (OGTT)
- Elevated haemoglobin A1c (HbA1c)

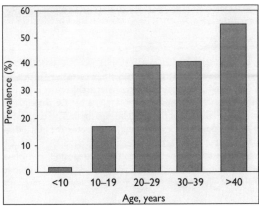

Figure 8.1 Prevalence of CFRD at the University of Minnesota by age group, in a population of more than 500 patients.

Elevated HbA1c was added as a diagnostic criterion for CFRD in 2010, with the caveat that low or normal HbA1c levels do not exclude the diagnosis of CFRD because levels tend to be spuriously low in CF. Inclusion of HbA1c elevation keeps the diagnostic criteria for CFRD in line with the ADA diagnostic criteria for other forms of diabetes.

8.2.2 **Diabetic status changes with time**

Over time, there may be considerable fluctuation in glucose tolerance in a given individual with CF. Insulin resistance in CF patients is often variable, dependent on changing infectious status, medications, and nutrition. Someone with CF who is diagnosed with diabetes during an infective exacerbation may return to glucose levels in the normal range weeks or months later, but will most likely become hyperglycaemic again during the next exacerbation. Once a person is diagnosed with CFRD, he or she always considered to have diabetes, even as hyperglycaemia waxes and wanes.

8.2.3 **Epidemiology**

The incidence and prevalence of glucose intolerance and CFRD in persons with CF is higher than in any other age-matched group. While it can occur at any age, CFRD prevalence clearly increases as patients get older. Young age does not preclude a diagnosis of CFRD; there are isolated case reports of infants with CFRD. The European Epidemiologic Registry of Cystic Fibrosis (ERCF) reported 5% and 13% prevalence in age groups 10–14 and 15–19 years, respectively. A prospective trial from Ireland reported similar prevalence figures: NGT–69%, IGT–14%, and CFRD–17% in the 10–19 years age group. At the University of Minnesota CF Center, diabetes was found in <5% of children aged 10 years and younger, 15–20% of adolescents, ~40% of those in their 20s and 30s, and >50% of those older than 40 years (see Figure 8.1), observations that are supported by those from several national registries.

8.3 **Pathophysiology**

The pathophysiology of CFRD is complex, and is related to physical destruction of islets as exocrine tissue is destroyed, genetic susceptibility, the influence of chronic inflammation and acute infection, malnutrition, and perhaps to the impact of the CF chloride channel on the beta cell itself (see Figure 8.2).

8.3.1 **Pancreas pathology**

Abnormal chloride channel function in CF results in thick viscous secretions causing obstructive damage to the exocrine pancreas, with progressive fibrosis and fatty infiltration. This results in disruption and destruction of islet architecture leading to loss of endocrine β-, α-, and pancreatic polypeptide cells. Thus, most CF patients, with or without diabetes, appear to have lost about half of their islet mass. The correlation between the degree of β-cell destruction and development of diabetes is poor, however, and postmortem studies have not shown a greater loss of islets in patients with CFRD compared to those with NGT. Islet amyloid polypeptide (IAPP) deposition, which is characteristic of T2D, was found on autopsy in 69% of CF patients with CFRD, while it was absent in those without diabetes. This suggests a common pathologic mechanism between CFRD and T2D.

CF β-cell dysfunction is not related to autoimmune disease. While there were some early reports suggesting the presence of diabetes autoantibodies in CFRD, a more definitive study demonstrated that the frequency of diabetes autoantibodies and HLA types associated with T1D are similar to that of the general population in patients with CFRD. Isolated case reports of autoantibody positive individuals with CFRD suggest there may be occasional patients with co-existing T1D.

Whether the basic CF chloride channel defect is directly involved in β-cell dysfunction in CF is uncertain. CFTR is expressed in β-cells, but its function there is unknown. It has been speculated that CF β-cell failure may be related to endoplasmic reticulum stress from retained abnormal CFTR protein, leading to apoptosis. A direct role for CFTR in insulin secretion has also been postulated, given interesting pilot data suggesting that correction of CFTR may increase insulin secretion.

8.3.2 **Genetics**

CFRD mainly occurs in people with CF mutations which produce severe disease and are associated with exocrine pancreatic insufficiency. A genetic association between CF and T2D is suggested by the increased prevalence of diabetes in monozygotic versus dizygotic twins with CF and an increased prevalence of CFRD in individuals with a family history of T2D. A possible link has been described between CFRD and T2D susceptibility genes, as well as genes associated with inflammation such as tumor necrosis factor, heat shock protein, and calpain 10. These findings have led to the hypothesis that while the primary pathologic defect in CFRD is partial loss of islets due to physical destruction, those subjects with underlying defects in insulin secretion or sensitivity may be more susceptible to diabetes because they are less able to compensate for reduced β-cell mass.

8.3.3 **The role of insulin deficiency**

The primary defect in CFRD is severe but not absolute insulin deficiency. Virtually all exocrine-insufficient patients with CF, with and without diabetes, have some degree of β-cell dysfunction. Fasting insulin and C-peptide concentrations may be normal, but there is delay and blunting of peak insulin secretion during a standard OGTT, where time to peak insulin secretion is 90–120 minutes compared to 30–60 minutes in healthy subjects. This effect is more pronounced with worsening glycaemic status. Delayed insulin secretion during the OGTT is related to loss of first phase insulin secretion, which is found even in CF patients with NGT.

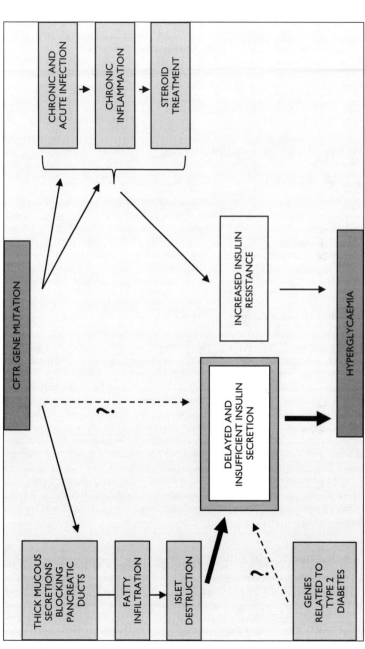

Figure 8.2 Possible mechanisms for abnormal glucose homeostasis in CF patients.

8.3.4 **The role of insulin resistance**

In CF patients without diabetes, insulin sensitivity has been reported as normal, increased, or decreased. These differences are most likely related to the acute state of health of the individual patient, since infection and inflammation influence insulin resistance. CF patients with diabetes have insulin resistance which is usually modest, including both decreased peripheral glucose uptake and poor insulin suppression of hepatic glucose production. For all CF patients, insulin resistance can become acutely severe during infectious exacerbations. Insulin resistance is not as important as insulin deficiency in the development of CFRD.

8.4 **Survival and prognosis**

8.4.1 **Mortality in CFRD**

The presence of diabetes was initially shown to be associated with worse lung function, poorer nutritional status, and decreased survival in persons with CF in North America and Europe, with a particularly negative impact on women. In the UK CF Registry, HbA1c >6.5% was associated with a threefold increase in the risk of death. However, longitudinal data have shown consistent improvement in survival and elimination of gender differences in mortality over the last 2 decades. This improvement has occurred in association with institution of routine OGTT screening which has led to early diagnosis, and with early institution of insulin therapy.

8.4.2 **Pre-diabetic morbidity**

Several studies have shown that an insidious decline in clinical status occurs in the years before the diagnosis of CFRD, in the insulin-insufficient, pre-diabetic state. In a prospective study, the decline in pulmonary function over 4 years was greatest in CF patients with diabetes, less in IGT, and least in patients with NGT. Pulmonary deterioration correlated with the degree of insulin deficiency at baseline. Others have also found that patients who secrete the least amount of insulin have the worst lung function and nutritional status. Given the known association between protein catabolism, malnutrition, and death in CF, and the potent anabolic effect of insulin, the nutritional impact of insulin insufficiency appears to be of greater consequence in CF than the metabolic impact of hyperglycaemia. This may result in clinical compromise long before glucose levels are high enough to qualify for a diagnosis of diabetes. This might be particularly relevant in growing children. In one study, the decline in BMI and lung function was more pronounced in those with younger onset CFRD, who were twice as likely to need oral nutritional supplements and four times more likely to require enteral feeding at the time of diabetes diagnosis compared to older subjects who developed diabetes.

8.5 **Complications of diabetes**

The primary purpose for establishing diagnoses is to identify expected outcomes and to inform treatment decisions. ADA and WHO diabetes diagnostic criteria have changed over time to reflect new information regarding the correlation between the level of hyperglycaemia and risk of microvascular complications in T1D and T2D. While these diabetes complications do occur in CFRD, the prevalence of retinopathy and nephropathy appears to be less than that found in other forms of diabetes and the conditions tend to be less severe. These complications are of lesser concern in CFRD than the impact of diabetes on death from pulmonary disease and malnutrition. For CF patients who have abnormal glucose tolerance which does not meet the threshold of severity required for a diabetes diagnosis, there are not sufficient data at present to determine a 'cut-off' point or a particular degree of hyperglycaemia and/or insulin insufficiency which confers added risk.

8.5.1 Microvascular complications

Diabetes microvascular complications occur in CFRD, and there are case reports of patients with significant morbidity such as blindness and renal failure. These tend to be the exception. In Denmark, 36% of patients with more than 10 years duration of diabetes had retinopathy. In a larger series of 285 CFRD patients, no CFRD FH- patient (up to 14 years' duration) had microvascular complications, while in CFRD FH+ complications were rare before 10 years' duration of disease. However, of the 39 subjects who had CFRD FH+ of more than 10 years' duration, microalbuminuria was found in 14%, retinopathy 16%, neuropathy 55%, and gastropathy 50%. These complications tended to be mild in nature. While the prevalence of diabetes microvascular complications appears to be lower in CFRD and the severity less than in other forms of diabetes, it remains important to screen for these complications since early detection can impact outcome.

Annual urine albumin screening and retinal exams are recommended for those diagnosed with CFRD with fasting hyperglycaemia for a duration of 5 years or more.

8.5.2 Macrovascular complications

Death from atherosclerotic cardiovascular disease has never been reported in CF, despite the fact that these patients are living longer. CF patients generally have low cholesterol concentrations, although isolated hypertriglyceridemia does occur, perhaps related to inflammation.

8.6 Clinical features of CFRD

8.6.1 Presentation

The median age of CFRD diagnosis is 18–24 years, although it can present at any age. It may present at a younger age in girls. CFRD develops insidiously and patients may be asymptomatic for years. In a large prospective Danish study of 191 patients, two-thirds of patients with CFRD were asymptomatic at the time of diagnosis.

Patients who have overt symptoms of hyperglycaemia on presentation (polyuria, polydipsia) have a relatively greater decline in pulmonary function and weight loss compared to those identified by routine screening. CFRD often first presents during situations where insulin resistance is increased, presumably by unmasking the underlying β-cell defect, such as with acute pulmonary infection, chronic severe lung disease, glucocorticoid therapy, high-carbohydrate food supplementation (oral, intravenous, or percutaneous gastrostomy tubes), and in association with transplantation. The incidence of CFRD is higher in those with CF liver disease. Diabetic ketoacidosis can occur but is rare, mostly likely because of the persistence of endogenous insulin secretion or because glucagon secretion is also impaired.

8.7 Screening for CFRD

Because CFRD is often clinically silent and because early intervention improves prognosis, routine screening for the disease is important. Hyperglycaemia may be intermittent, and normal fasting or random glucose concentrations do not exclude a diagnosis of diabetes. In addition, blood glucose levels in response to meals at home or in response to a mixed-meal study are often better than those obtained during OGTT, probably because of the beneficial effects of endogenous incretin secretion. Annual routine OGTT screening is recommended for all patients ≥10 years not known to have CFRD, because the results have been shown to correlate with long-term prognosis and with response to therapy. Some centres recommend that screening begin as early as age 6. More intensive screening (additional OGTT, blood glucose monitoring, CGM) should be considered in the following circumstances:

- symptoms of diabetes in CF patients of all ages (polyuria, polydipsia)
- failure to gain or maintain weight despite nutritional intervention
- poor growth velocity
- delayed progression of puberty
- unexplained chronic decline in pulmonary function
- during pulmonary exacerbations
- during systemic glucocorticoid therapy
- during supplemental enteral feedings
- the presence of CF liver disease
- pre/post major surgery
- pregnancy (ideally pre-conception, otherwise as soon as the pregnancy is detected)

8.7.1 **Oral glucose tolerance test**

The OGTT is the standard screening test for CFRD (see Table 8.3). CFRD FH- can only be detected by OGTT. Nearly two-thirds of adults with a diagnosis of CFRD do not have fasting hyperglycaemia. It is important to identify these individuals because they are at high risk for both significant lung function decline and for progression to fasting hyperglycaemia, and because insulin therapy has been shown to improve nutritional status in this population.

There are emerging data that glucose levels mid-OGTT may be more predictive of declining nutritional status or lung function than the 2-hour glucose level. It is important to note

Table 8.3 OGTT protocol
The patient should be at their clinical baseline at the time of testing
The patient should not be receiving systemic glucocorticoids unless this is a chronic state
The patient is fasted for at least 8 hours
The test is performed in the morning
Time 0—blood is taken in a fluoride oxalate tube, and clearly labelled with time of testing
A glucose load is ingested over not more than 5 minutes: Adults: equivalent to 75 g anhydrous glucose in a total fluid volume of 250–300 ml   Children: 1.75 g glucose per kg bodyweight, to a maximum of 75 g
Timing for the tests starts at start of ingestion
At a minimum, a second glucose sample is taken after 120 minutes. Samples may also be collected at 30, 60, and 90 minutes since emerging data suggests these values give important prognostic information
The patient should avoid exercise or exertion during the test

that an OGTT with glucose measured at all time points (0, 30, 60, 90, and 120 minutes), is necessary to diagnose indeterminate glycaemia.

While most centers do not start OGTT screening of children before the age of 10 years, a study from the University of Minnesota found that that 42% of children with CF age 6–9 years already had abnormal glucose tolerance with either IGT or indeterminate glycaemia (Ode et al., 2010). Those with abnormal glucose tolerance were at high risk for progression to diabetes as they entered puberty. Contrary to reports of severe malnutrition and worse lung function in youths diagnosed with CFRD at other centers, these young patients at the University of Minnesota did not differ in weight or lung function from their non-diabetic CF peers, suggesting the benefits of early OGTT detection of diabetes risk.

8.7.2 Haemoglobin A1c

HbA1c (the percentage of haemoglobin that is glycosylated, reflecting recent average blood glucose levels) has been shown by several investigators to be unreliable in the diagnosis of CFRD. Spuriously low HbA1c is hypothesized, but not proven, to be related to increased red blood cell turnover due to inflammation. An elevated HbA1c (>6.5%) is evidence of hyperglycaemia, but a normal HbA1c does not exclude it.

8.7.3 Continuous glucose monitoring

Continuous glucose monitoring (CGM) has been validated and proven to be useful in children and adolescents with CFRD, where it can help guide safe and effective insulin therapy. Its role in CF patients who do not have diabetes is less clear. It is well known that post-prandial glycaemic abnormalities exist in patients with CF long before OGTT results move from NGT to IGT, but to-date the clinical significance of these brief elevations in glucose excursion remains unclear. Some investigators have shown greater lung function decline in individuals associated with increased periods of hyperglycaemia on CGM or greater risk of glucose tolerance deterioration. Figure 8.3 shows CGM recordings demonstrating variations in glucose excursion in 3 different CF patients evaluated at home under usual conditions of diet and activity. Work remains to be done to determine the correlation between CGM findings and pulmonary and nutritional outcomes in CF, in order to define the point at which insulin therapy should be considered.

8.8 Treatment of CFRD

8.8.1 Medical nutritional therapy

Malnutrition is well-known to be associated with poor growth, pubertal delay, diminished lung function, and early death in CF. CF consensus guidelines stress the importance of a high-calorie, high-fat diet. These recommendations are the same for CF patients who develop diabetes (see Table 8.4). Thus, it is important to keep in mind that the diet recommended for persons with CFRD is very different from that prescribed to persons with T1D and T2D, and CF-specific guidelines must be followed.

8.8.2 Insulin therapy

At present, insulin is the only recommended medical therapy for CFRD (see Box 8.1). The general principles of insulin therapy are presented in Table 8.5. Many different regimens are possible depending on individual patient needs. As in other forms of diabetes, effective basal-bolus therapy can be accomplished with an insulin pump, or with a combination of long-acting basal insulin and rapid-acting insulin to cover carbohydrates and correct hyperglycaemia. Insulin therapy stabilizes lung function and improves nutritional status in

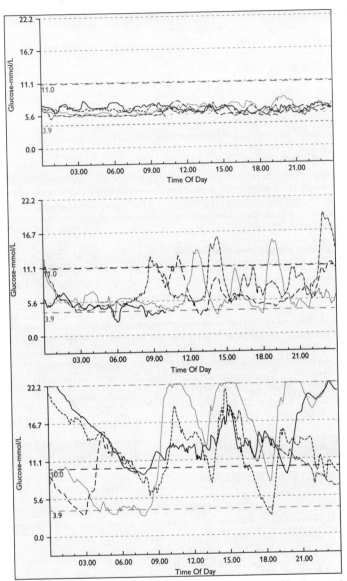

Figure 8.3 Examples of continuous glucose monitoring readings in individual CF patients ranging from normal (top, all interstitial glucose measurements less than 8 mmol/L), to post-prandial hyperglycaemia (middle) to severe hyperglycaemia (bottom). Traces represent 4 consecutive days' measurements overlayed, with time on the x axis (24 hrs).

Table 8.4 Medical nutrition therapy

	Types 1 and 2 Diabetes	CFRD
Calories	≤100% of normal for age and gender—often have to watch or restrict calories to prevent overweight	Usually require 120–150% (or more) of normal caloric intake for age and gender to prevent underweight
Fat	<35% of total energy	40% of total energy
Total carbohydrate	45–60% total energy	45–50% total energy
Fibre	No quantitative recommendation, but encouraged due to beneficial effects	Encouraged in the well nourished, but in poorly nourished patients may compromise energy intake
Protein	10–20% of total energy; not >1 g per kg body weight	200% of reference nutrient intake
Salt	Low intake, ≤6g /day	Increased requirement: unrestricted intake

Box 8.1 CFRD treatment summary

CFRD patients die from chronic, inflammatory lung disease, and thus treatment of the CF takes precedence and follows the usual recommendations for the CF population.

Diabetes management should be modified according to the individual's needs.

As for all persons with CF, the energy requirements are at least 150% of normal, with a goal of about 40% fat, 20% protein, and 40% carbohydrates. Typically these patients eat at least 3 meals and 3 snacks per day. Pancreatic supplements are essential at each meal and snack.

Insulin is the only recommended treatment for CFRD. In CF, where adequate nutritional status is necessary for survival, the anabolic effect of insulin is likely to be even more important than its effect on glycaemia.

The insulin regimen should be adjusted to match the diet rather than asking patients to change their diet to fit an insulin regimen. This generally requires carbohydrate counting and matching insulin to carbohydrate intake.

Insulin can be delivered by multiple daily injections or through insulin pump therapy.

Checking glucose levels with home blood glucose monitoring or CGM is important.

Self-care education programs promote independence and encourage patients to adjust diet and insulin doses themselves.

patients with CFRD. In contrast to other forms of diabetes, the most important aspect of insulin therapy in CF may not be restoration of normoglycaemia. Because of the relationship between nutritional status and survival in this population, the anabolic effects of insulin may be the most critical aspect of therapy. Thus, the goal is to provide as high an insulin dose as the patient can safely tolerate.

8.8.3 Oral diabetes agents

Oral diabetes agents are currently not recommended in CFRD. A Cochrane review identified 19 studies with 24 references, but none were randomized controlled trials other than

Table 8.5 General principles of insulin therapy in CFRD	
Total insulin dose	• The average total daily insulin dose in CF is 0.4–0.5 units/kg/day in adolescents and adults, but this varies between patients and, in individuals, can vary from day to day based on overall health • When well, most CF patients are relatively easy to manage, similar to the honeymoon phase of T1D • When ill, they can be tremendously insulin resistant • The goal is to provide as much insulin as the patient can safely tolerate, to restore the patient to an anabolic state
Meal coverage	• A common starting dose is 0.5–1.0 units rapid-acting insulin per 15 grams carbohydrate • The dose is adjusted by increments of 0.5 units per 15 grams carbohydrate to achieve 2-hr post-prandial blood glucose goals • Insulin pens or syringes that deliver half units may be needed • For very young patients or those who are unsure of what they will eat due to nausea or gastroparesis, the dose can be given right after the meal, or part of the dose given before and part after the meal
Correction dose	• Pre-meal correction can be started at 0.5–1 unit rapid-acting insulin for every 2.8 mmol/L (50 mg/dl) above target and adjusted as needed
Basal insulin	• Basal insulin can be started at 0.25 units per kg body weight per 24 hours, and adjusted based on the fasting glucose level • Patients with CFRD without fasting hyperglycaemia may be managed with pre-meal insulin alone, or with basal alone (depending on patient factors, including eating habits)
Overnight feed	• For an 8–10 hr overnight feed, start at a total dose of 0.5–1 unit per 15 grams carbohydrate, divided as half intermediate release insulin (NPH) + half regular insulin (regular insulin covers the first half and NPH the second half of the feeding); glucose levels 4 hrs into the feeding and at the end are used to adjust the insulin dose

the CFRDT Trial. The insulin secretagogue repaglinide increased endogenous insulin concentrations but was less effective than rapid-acting insulin at regulating post-prandial hyperglycaemia in an acute experimental setting, and was not able to produce sustained weight gain in individuals with CFRD FH- in the CFRDT trial.

Concern has been expressed over the use of sulphonylureas in CFRD because of evidence that they bind to and inhibit CFTR, and because early experience suggested problems with hypoglycaemia with these agents in CF. Agents that reduce insulin resistance are unlikely to be effective as a single therapy in CFRD, since insulin resistance is not a major aetiological factor. The gastrointestinal side effects of metformin such as nausea, diarrhoea, and abdominal discomfort are unacceptable to most people with CF. Thiazolidinediones have been associated with osteoporosis which calls into question the use of these drugs in CF. There are no data on the clinical use of incretins in CF, although those that decrease gastric emptying would not be expected to be good candidates for this population.

8.8.4 Inpatient management of CFRD

During acute illness, patients with CF are at high risk of developing hyperglycaemia. There are no specific studies of the benefits of maintaining euglycaemia in hospitalized CF patients, but data from other populations have been extrapolated to suggest that intensive insulin therapy may be beneficial in this setting. Insulin requirements are often quite large during acute illness. CFRD patients who regularly receive insulin require far more, often up to 4 times their usual dose. It is important to remember that the insulin dose must be aggressively reduced as the patient improves.

8.8.5 **New treatment options for CF may impact CFRD**

Several exciting new drugs are in the pipeline to 'correct' or 'potentiate' the defective CFTR chloride channel (see Chapter 13). The first of these to be approved for clinical application is ivacaftor (see Chapter 4). A small pilot study has shown improved insulin secretion in response to ivacaftor therapy, suggesting the intriguing possibility that CFTR is involved in insulin secretion and that correction of CFTR might prevent or ameliorate CFRD. Similar drugs in development are aimed at the general CF population, and may ultimately have a profound effect on the risk of developing diabetes.

8.9 **Treatment of CF patients with abnormal glucose tolerance**

Small, uncontrolled studies suggest that patients with IGT might benefit from insulin therapy. However, there are no definitive data on the benefits of insulin therapy for CF patients with milder forms of abnormal glucose tolerance. This has been identified as a high-priority research question.

References

Blackman SM, Commander CW, Watson C, et al. Genetic modifiers of cystic fibrosis-related diabetes. *Diabetes* 2013;62:3627–35.

Dobson L, Sheldon CD, Hattersley AT. Conventional measures underestimate glycaemia in CF patients. *Diabet Med* 2004;21:691–6.

Frohnert B, Ode KL, Moran A, et al. Impaired fasting glucose in cystic fibrosis. *Diabetes Care* 2010;33:2660–4.

Moran A, Becker D, Casella SJ, et al. Epidemiology, pathophysiology and prognostic implications of CFRD: a technical review. *Diabetes Care* 2010;33:2677–83.

Moran A, Brunzell C, Cohen RC, et al. Clinical care guidelines for CFRD: recommendations from the Cystic Fibrosis Foundation, the American Diabetes Association and the Pediatric Endocrine Society. *Diabetes Care* 2010;33:2697–708

Moran A, Dunitz J, Nathan B, et al. Cystic fibrosis related diabetes: current trends in prevalence, incidence and mortality. *Diabetes Care* 2009;32:1626–31.

Moran A, Pekow P, Grover P, et al. Insulin therapy to improve BMI in cystic fibrosis related diabetes without fasting hyperglycemia: results of the Cystic Fibrosis Related Diabetes Therapy trial. *Diabetes Care* 2009;32:1783–8.

Onady GM, Stolfi A. Insulin and oral agents for managing cystic fibrosis-related diabetes. *Cochrane Database Syst Rev* 2013, Jul 26;7:CD004730.

O'Riordan SMP, Robinson PD, Donaghue KC, et al. ISPAD clinical practice consensus guidelines 2008: management of cystic fibrosis-related diabetes. *Pediatric Diabetes* 2008;9:338–44.

O'Riordan SM, Hindmarsh P, Hill NR, et al. Validation of continuous glucose monitoring in children and adolescents with cystic fibrosis: a prospective cohort study. *Diabetes Care* 2009; 32:1020–2.

Chapter 9

Metabolic and musculoskeletal effects of cystic fibrosis

Uta Hill, Jane Ashbrook, and Charles Haworth

> **Key points**
>
> - 10 – 25% of adults with cystic fibrosis (CF) have low bone mineral density (BMD)
> - Risk factors for low BMD include CFTR genotype, male gender, low body mass index (BMI), pulmonary infection/systemic inflammation, pubertal delay, hypogonadism, oral corticosteroid use, vitamin D insufficiency, and vitamin K insufficiency
> - Approximately 10% of adults with CF develop a non-erosive episodic arthritis characterized by painful swelling of the hands, wrists, knees, and ankles
> - Impaired growth in CF is associated with nutritional deficiency, lung infection, and systemic inflammation
> - Urinary incontinence is a significant problem for girls and women with CF. It is best managed by experienced physiotherapy input to retrain pelvic muscle responses during coughing

9.1 Osteoporosis

9.1.1 Introduction

Osteoporosis is a progressive systemic skeletal disease characterized by low bone mass and micro-architectural deterioration of bone tissue, with a consequent increase in bone fragility and susceptibility to fracture. Risk factors for osteoporosis in the general population include a parental history of hip fracture, a prior history of osteoporotic fracture, low body mass index, glucocorticoid use, smoking, high alcohol intake, and secondary causes of osteoporosis such as rheumatoid arthritis, hypogonadism, prolonged immobility, organ transplantation, type 1 diabetes, hyperthyroidism, gastrointestinal disease, chronic liver disease, and chronic obstructive pulmonary disease. The risk of fracture increases with decreasing bone mineral density. Observational (non-CF) population-based studies suggest that the risk of fracture approximately doubles for each standard deviation reduction in bone mineral density.

Dual-energy X-ray absorptiometry (DXA) is the most widely endorsed methodology for measuring bone mineral density and involves a very low effective radiation dose (<1 mSv per site). For comparison, the effective dose of a chest X-ray is 20 mSv. Bone density results are presented as Z scores (the standard deviation score from the mean of an age- and sex-matched control population) or as T scores (the standard deviation score from the mean of a sex-matched control population at peak bone mass).

9.1.2 **Osteoporotic fractures**

Fracture rates are increased in CF patients compared to the general population and most commonly affect the ribs and vertebral bodies (see Figures 9.1 and 9.2). These are clinically important as they are painful, prevent effective airway clearance, and can lead to worsening lung infection. Rib fractures can also cause pneumothorax.

Fractures of the proximal femur usually require surgical intervention, which is problematic in patients with advanced lung disease. A history of osteoporotic fracture may also be a relative contra-indication to lung transplant listing.

9.1.3 **Bone mineral density measurements**

Dual energy X-ray absorptiometry (DXA) provides an areal (2-dimensional) assessment rather than a volumetric (3-dimensional) assessment of BMD. The interpretation of areal BMD poses major challenges in healthy children due to changes in bone size related to age and puberty, and in children with chronic diseases (such as CF) in whom poor growth and delayed puberty adversely affect bone size. DXA therefore often overestimates deficits in BMD in individuals with short stature/small bones. Various corrections have been proposed such as correcting for height, pubertal stage, and body composition, but these are usually only used in research settings. Consequently, BMD reference data are less reliable for paediatric, adolescent, and young adult populations than adult populations.

The UK Cystic Fibrosis Trust Bone Mineralisation Working Group recommends that BMD values should be expressed as Z scores in premenopausal women and in men under the age

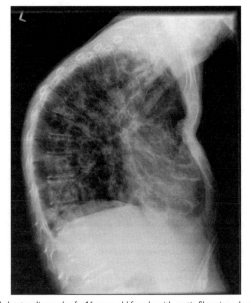

Figure 9.1 Lateral chest radiograph of a 16-year-old female with cystic fibrosis and severe lung disease and osteoporotic fractures of the sternum and vertebral bodies of C6 and C7.

Latzin P, Griese M, Hermanns M, and Kramer B. Images in Thorax: Sternal fracture with fatal outcome in cystic fibrosis. *Thorax* 2005;60:616.

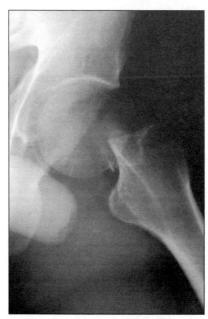

Figure 9.2 Fractured neck of femur in a 21-year-old man with cystic fibrosis and osteoporosis.
Haworth CS, Selby PL, Webb AK, and Adams JE. Osteoporosis in adults with cystic fibrosis. *J Royal Soc Med* 1998;91(Suppl. 34):14–18.

of 50 years, and as T scores thereafter. It is also recommended that the term 'CF-related low bone mineral density' be applied to children or adults with CF who have a BMD Z score below -2, with the caveat that Z scores may be unreliable in individuals of small body size.

Cross-sectional studies suggest that BMD is normal or near normal in well-nourished children with CF who have well-preserved lung function. However, deficits in BMD are apparent in adolescents and are even more evident in young adults, such that 10–25% have low bone density (defined as having a Z score <-2). Longitudinal BMD studies suggest inadequate bone mass accrual in children and adolescents with CF. In addition, young adults with CF show rates of bone loss of around 2% in the proximal femur, suggesting that there may also be premature bone loss in early adult life (see Figure 9.3).

9.1.4 **Risk factors for low BMD**

The risk factors for low BMD in CF are outlined in Table 9.1.

Genotype

CFTR has been identified in human osteoblasts and osteoclasts. Although the functional significance of this finding is unclear, patients with the ΔF508 mutation have lower bone density than patients with other genotypes, and ΔF508 homozygotes have higher bone turnover than non-ΔF508 homozygotes, which suggests that CFTR may influence bone cell activity.

Gender difference

Several studies have also reported that low BMD is more common in males than females, although the cause of this association is unclear. The gender difference may reflect

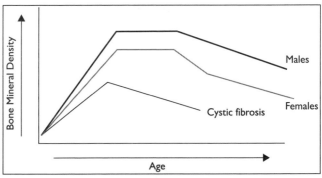

Figure 9.3 Change in bone mineral density over time in healthy males and females; and change in bone mineral density in cystic fibrosis where peak bone mass may occur early and be followed by premature bone loss.

Table 9.1 Risk factors for low bone mineral density in CF
CFTR genotype
Male gender
CF disease severity
Low forced expiratory volume in 1 second
Low body mass index
High intravenous antibiotic requirement
C-reactive protein
Reduced levels of weight bearing exercise
Pancreatic insufficiency
Malnutrition
Malabsorption of fat-soluble vitamins
Vitamin D insufficiency
Vitamin K insufficiency
Calcium malabsorption
Corticosteroid use
Diabetes
Liver disease
Pubertal delay and hypogonadism

the protective effects of female sex hormones on BMD or relative hypogonadism in the males.

Disease severity

There is a clear association between low BMD and CF disease severity. It is thought that increased expression of pro-inflammatory cytokines due to acute and chronic lung infection leads to increased osteoclast activity in CF. This is supported by the observation that biochemical markers of bone resorption are increased at the start of pulmonary exacerbations and reduce following intravenous antibiotic treatment.

Vitamin deficiencies

Vitamin D deficiency, defined as a 25-hydroxyvitamin D level <5 ng/ml, is associated with osteomalacia, a condition that leads to low BMD due to an increase in the proportion of non-mineralized bone tissue. Vitamin D insufficiency, defined as a 25-hydroxyvitamin D level <30 ng/ml (approx. 70 nmol/L), was found in approximately 75% of patients with cystic fibrosis despite routine daily supplementation with 800 iu ergocalciferol. Vitamin D insufficiency is associated with a relative hyperparathyroid state and induces osteoclastic bone resorption. Serum parathyroid hormone (PTH) concentrations should be measured in conjunction with 25-hydroxyvitamin D concentrations when determining vitamin D status in patients with CF. It is important to note that 25-hydroxyvitamin D concentrations fluctuate through the seasons according to the amount of solar exposure. Thus, the time of year and recent travel history should be considered when interpreting vitamin D results.

Vitamin K is an essential cofactor in the carboxylation of osteocalcin, the main non-collagenous protein in bone. In its carboxylated form, osteocalcin binds to hydroxyapatite and is thought to have a role in the regulation of bone formation. Vitamin K insufficiency leads to increased levels of undercarboxylated osteocalcin, which is likely to adversely affect bone formation as it binds less effectively to hydroxyapatite. Unlike vitamins A, D, and E, vitamin K is not routinely supplemented in most CF centres unless the prothrombin time is increased. As the liver is more efficient in utilizing vitamin K, a prolonged prothrombin time is a late marker of vitamin K deficiency.

Medications

Glucocorticoids suppress bone formation by osteoblasts, suppress sex steroids in men and women, and increase bone resorption in the early phase of steroid therapy. Glucocorticoids also reduce calcium absorption from the gut and increase calcium excretion in the kidney, which in turn lead to increased parathyroid activity. Several studies have shown a clear association between low BMD and oral corticosteroid use in CF.

9.1.5 Screening for low bone mineral density

The optimal age from which to start performing DXA screening for low BMD in CF is unclear. Some authorities suggest screening from about the age of 10 years, whereas others suggest performing DXA scans after peak height has been achieved to minimize the effect of bone size.

DXA scans should be repeated every 1–3 years depending on the results of the test and the clinical well-being of the patient. Serial scans allow the identification of peak bone mass, following which antiresorptive treatments can be added if required. In addition, chest X-rays should routinely be examined for the presence of fragility fractures affecting the ribs and vertebral bodies.

9.1.6 Strategies to prevent low BMD

An approach to optimizing bone health is outlined in Table 9.2.

Nutrition

The CF-centre dietitian has a central role in optimizing bone health in children and adults with CF. Optimizing growth and lean body mass are fundamental to achieving this goal, and specialist knowledge of appropriate calorific intake and pancreatic enzyme replacement therapy is required.

Table 9.2 Strategies to prevent low bone mineral density in CF
Nutritional factors
Optimize growth and lean body mass
Optimize calcium intake
Correct vitamin D and vitamin K insufficiency
Endocrine factors
Correct pubertal delay and hypogonadism
Optimize control of CF related diabetes
Systemic Inflammation
Optimize control of lung infection
Encourage weight-bearing exercise
Minimize corticosteroid use

Vitamin supplementation

North American guidelines advocate achieving 25-hydroxyvitamin D levels of >30 ng/ml (70 nmol/L), based on the finding that PTH levels rise when the 25-hydroxyvitamin D level is <30 ng/ml. Achieving and then sustaining this level over the long term can be difficult in practice, even with high-dose vitamin D replacement regimens.

Most centres prescribe between 800–1600 iu vitamin D/day to CF patients over the age of 12 years and add combined calcium + vitamin D supplements if the 25-hydroxyvitamin D level is inadequate. As vitamin A is often combined with vitamin D in supplements, care must be taken to prevent vitamin A toxicity if dosing is increased in an attempt to boost 25-hydroxyvitamin D levels. Alternative strategies include using high-dose colecalciferol (20–40 000 iu weekly) or cautious ultraviolet B exposure.

Calcium intake should usually be 1300–1500 mg/day from the age of 8 years. Care should be taken to calculate the amount of calcium in oral supplements and overnight feeds, in addition to that taken in the regular diet.

Vitamin K supplements are not routinely prescribed to CF patients at present, although practice is changing. Some centres prescribe AquADEKs®, a CF-specific multivitamin preparation that contains vitamin K, and some centres prescribe phytomenadione 5–10 mg daily from the age of 7 years.

Endocrine and hormonal surveillance

The UK Cystic Fibrosis Trust Bone Mineralisation Working Group recommends that pubertal development should be assessed in girls from around the age of 9 years and boys from around the age of 11 years. A morning serum testosterone should be measured annually in adult males and a menstrual history should be taken annually in adolescent/adult females to screen for hypogonadism. An endocrine referral should be made in patients with delayed puberty or hypogonadism. When indicated, glucocorticoid treatment should be kept to a minimum.

Other therapies

An individualized exercise programme should be developed for each patient by the CF specialist physiotherapist to optimize levels of weight-bearing activity.

Treatments to minimize lung infection/systemic inflammation should be implemented.

Advice, where necessary, should be provided on the adverse effects of smoking and alcohol on bone health.

9.1.7 **Management of low BMD**

The standard measures outlined in Table 9.2 should be applied to all patients with low BMD.

Bisphosphonates are analogues of inorganic pyrophosphate and inhibit bone resorption. Randomized controlled trials of oral (daily and weekly regimens) and intravenous bisphosphonates show that bisphosphonate treatment leads to significant increases BMD in adults with CF. However, none of the bisphosphonate trials in CF were powered to detect changes in fracture prevalence.

Intermittent intravenous administration of bisphosphonates overcomes the poor gastrointestinal absorption, and the potential oesophageal complications, of oral bisphosphonates. Bisphosphonate use is associated with severe bone pain after the first 1–3 doses in a proportion of patients with CF. Pain is observed less commonly in patients starting bisphosphonate treatment after a course of intravenous antibiotics and in patients taking oral corticosteroids, suggesting that lung infection/inflammation is a risk factor for developing bone pain. The pain tends to last up to 72 hours and can be sufficiently severe to require opiate analgesia.

The UK Cystic Fibrosis Trust Bone Mineralisation Working Group recommends that bisphosphonate treatment in adults should be considered when:

- A patient has sustained a fragility fracture
- The lumbar spine or total hip or femoral neck BMD Z score is <−2, and there is evidence of significant bone loss (>4% per year) on serial DXA measurements despite implementation of the general measures to improve bone health
- A patient is starting a prolonged (greater than 3 months) course of oral glucocorticoid treatment and has a BMD Z score <−1.5
- A patient is listed for or has received a solid organ transplant and has a BMD Z score <−1.5

Bisphosphonates are contra-indicated in pregnancy and so females of childbearing age should be counselled before starting treatment. Bisphosphonates should also not be prescribed in patients with vitamin D insufficiency. It is usual practice to prescribe calcium + vitamin D supplements in patients prescribed bisphosphonates. Bone densitometry should be performed approximately 12 months after starting bisphosphonate treatment to assess efficacy.

9.2 **Arthropathy and vasculitis**

9.2.1 **Arthropathy and musculoskeletal disorders**

Cystic fibrosis-related arthropathy (CFA) and hypertrophic osteoarthropathy (HOA) are two more common and well-described forms of joint disease in CF. Gout has also been noted in adult CF patients.

Approximately 9% of CF adults develop CFA which describes an asymmetric, non-erosive mono- or polyarthritis involving knees, ankles, wrists, elbows, or shoulders. Typically, joints become painful and stiff over 12–24 hours and this persists for up to 1 week. Associated features include a skin rash similar to erythema nodosum and fever. Radiography of involved joints is usually normal without evidence of joint destruction. The aetiology of CFA is unknown but several theories have been proposed. Chronic pulmonary infection may predispose to circulating immune complexes or the induction of autoantibodies due to cross-reactive antigens which can lead to joint inflammation. Treatment consists principally of non-steroidal anti-inflammatory agents and antibiotics for pulmonary exacerbation if present. Oral glucocorticoids are only used in refractory cases given the associated toxicity.

HOA in CF is less common than CFA with an estimated prevalence of 7% in the adult CF population and is characterized by periostitis at the distal end of long bones. Large joints (wrists, ankles, knees) are involved and symptoms are usually more florid during pulmonary exacerbations. Radiography of affected joints typically shows periosteal proliferation but the onset of these changes may be delayed relative to symptoms. Management includes non-steroidal anti-inflammatory agents for pain relief and antibiotics to reduce bacterial load.

The role of disease-modifying anti-rheumatic drugs (DMARDs) in CF patients with arthropathy has been the subject of a recent Cochrane review. Disappointingly, the authors could not identify any randomized trials but only 3 case reports and series describing the use of agents such as sulfasalazine, sodium aurothiomalate, methotrexate, or leflunomide in patients with CFA. Treatment success was limited either by further disease progression or the considerable side effect profile of the DMARDs. In refractory cases a limited trial of therapy may be indicated.

The prevalence of gout in adult CF patients has been estimated to be 2.5% (vs 1% in non-CF cohorts). Affected CF patients presented with acute monoarthritis affecting the great toe, foot, or ankle joints, typical of classical gout. Hyperuricaemia was also reported in approximately 30% of asymptomatic CF adults, significantly greater than the non-CF population. A possible explanation of hyperuricaemia in CF patients is excessive ingestion of pancreatic enzyme supplements which contain high levels of purines. It is therefore advisable to review the intake of pancreatic enzymes in CF patients with gout. Asymptomatic mild hyperuricaemia, however, does not usually require treatment.

Back pain and associated musculoskeletal disorders are common in CF. Abnormal posture characterised by kyphosis due to reduced BMD accompanied by a 'hunched flexed' posture in the context of hyperinflation and coughing are widely reported in adults with CF. This posture causes an imbalance in activity of the abdominal, pelvic, and spinal muscles, and alters the stresses placed on the spine, shoulder, and pelvic girdles resulting in a predisposition to painful disorders. Spinal stability is compromised further when respiratory drive is increased and these muscles forego their postural role to increase the work of breathing.

Regular postural assessment is advisable for individuals with CF. Exercises to maintain spinal mobility and muscle strength can improve posture and help to prevent deterioration of spinal position (see Figure 9.4). In cases where pain is present or spinal kyphosis is fixed, involvement of a musculoskeletal physiotherapist is recommended.

9.2.2 **Vasculitis**

Cutaneous vasculitis is occasionally seen in patients with episodic arthropathy and is thought to relate to bacterial infection and immune complex formation. The rash is most commonly petechial and usually affects the feet and lower limbs. Erythema nodosum can also occur. Anti-neutrophil cytoplasmic antibodies against bacterial-/permeability-increasing protein are often present. Treatment is with oral corticosteroids and antibiotics to reduce bacterial load. Vasculitis can also affect the bowel, kidneys, and central nervous system in CF, although this is extremely rare.

9.3 **Growth**

Impaired growth in CF is associated with nutritional deficiencies, lung infection, and systemic inflammation. It is thought that pro-inflammatory cytokines such as IL-6 and TNFα reduce sensitivity to growth hormone and decrease insulin-like growth factor secretion.

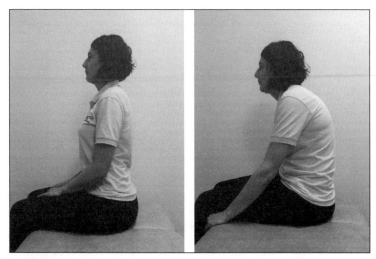

Figure 9.4 Illustration of normal upright sitting posture (left), and an example of an increased thoracic kyphosis commonly seen in CF (right).

Height and weight are often reduced in prepubertal children with CF and reduced height velocity is an early indicator of CF lung disease. Historical data also suggest that pubertal development is delayed in people with CF and is related to the degree of nutritional and lung function impairment. However, recent studies report normal pubertal progression as indicated by clinical pubertal staging and age at menarche, presumably reflecting improved health in childhood and adolescence.

Adult height is within the normal range for most individuals, but the mean height of adults with CF remains reduced compared to the general population.

Oral and inhaled corticosteroids may lead to impaired growth by suppressing growth hormone secretion. Relative insulin deficiency and the development of CF-related diabetes may adversely affect growth.

Growth may be enhanced by optimising control of lung infection, optimizing nutritional parameters, treating insulin deficiency, and by minimizing corticosteroid exposure. Neonatal screening and earlier diagnosis may also lead to improved growth in CF. Recombinant human growth hormone may be used to increase height, weight, lean body mass, and bone mineral content in prepubertal children with CF, but requires specialist endocrinology input.

9.4 **Urinary incontinence**

Urinary incontinence (UI) has now been recognized worldwide as a significant problem for girls and women with CF. It is defined as involuntary leakage of urine on exertion, or during manoeuvres such as sneezing or coughing, by the International Society of Continence. There are few literature reports of UI in men, and it remains very rare in this group. The patient-reported prevalence of UI ranges from 19–49% in girls with CF versus 8–13% in healthy teenagers, and from 30–69% in female CF patients versus 8–35% in healthy women. Coughing is recognized by the majority of patients as the major precipitant of urinary leakage; sneezing, laughing, exercise, and performing spirometry are reported as other precipitants. Typically, the amount of urinary leakage is small. During pulmonary exacerbations however, 49% of patients mention having to 'change underwear', and 22% report 'leakage down the legs'. Urinary leakage clearly has a significant negative impact on the quality of patients' lives. Girls and adolescents in particular may be very upset by incontinence and can take drastic measures, such as reducing fluid intake and avoiding leaving the house. As urinary leakage is often exacerbated during airway clearance exercises and spirometry, these may be avoided by patients, thereby further compromising the management of their lung disease.

The pathophysiology of UI in CF is multifactorial. Predisposing factors are increased intra-abdominal pressure secondary to frequent prolonged coughing, constipation, and inadequate pelvic floor function. Urinary continence during expectoration depends on a complex interaction of the muscles of the pelvic floor and the abdominal cavity. Prior to a cough, the diaphragm descends during inspiration, increasing intra-abdominal pressure. In response, the pelvic floor muscles contract to maintain urethral closure. This is followed by strong abdominal wall contraction during expiration to generate an effective cough. Timely contraction of the pelvic floor is therefore crucial to maintenance of continence during raised intra-abdominal pressure. In CF, however, increased frequency and severity of coughing, especially during exacerbations, exert considerable stress on the pelvic floor which may fail to contract appropriately. Studies have shown greater prevalence of UI in women who cough more and have a lower FEV_1.

Constipation, common in CF, is another risk factor for the development of UI. Distension of the rectum and colon secondary to impacted fecal material exerts pressure on the bladder and prolonged straining stretches the pelvic floor and weakens the musculature. This stretching during bowel movements can be lessened by raising the feet up onto a stool or hugging a knee into the chest, thereby altering the angle of the pelvis and reducing the pressure exerted on the pelvic floor and bladder.

Management of UI in CF patients has to-date been the subject of only a few small studies. The UK CF Trust recommends referral to experienced physiotherapists for assessment of incontinence and appropriate pelvic floor training exercises. Bladder management strategies can be put in place to help reduce the impact of stress UI. These include maintaining a good fluid balance throughout the day, reducing caffeine intake in food and drinks, and avoiding going to the toilet 'just in case'. The 'Knack' manoeuvre is a volitional pelvic floor muscle contraction that has been shown immediately to reduce leakage during activities of expected stress UI. Young females with CF should be taught the Knack as a preventative measure during activities where excessive stress is placed on the bladder and pelvic floor, such as coughing, spirometry, and airway clearance. More severe cases may benefit from gynaecological referral and consideration of trans-vaginal urethroplasty.

References

Aris RM, on behalf of the Cystic Fibrosis Foundation Consensus Bone Health Group. Guide to bone health and disease in cystic fibrosis. *J Clin Endocrinol Metab* 2005;90:1888–96.

Bone Mineralisation in Cystic Fibrosis. Report of the UK Cystic Fibrosis Trust Bone Mineralisation Working Group. February 2007.

Buntain HM, Schluter PJ, Bell SC, et al. Controlled longitudinal study of bone mass accrual in children and adolescents with cystic fibrosis. *Thorax* 2006;61:146–54.

Dodd ME, Langmann H. Urinary incontinence in cystic fibrosis. *J R Soc Med* 2005;98(Suppl. 45): 28–36.

Haworth CS, Selby PL, Webb AK, et al. Inflammatory related changes in bone mineral content in adults with cystic fibrosis. *Thorax* 2004;59:613–17.

Horsley A, Helm J, Brennan A, et al. Gout and hyperuricaemia in adults with cystic fibrosis. *J R Soc Med* 2011: S36–S39.

Miller JM, Sampselle C, Ashton-Miller J, et al. Clarification and confirmation of the Knack maneuver: the effect of volitional pelvic floor muscle contraction to pre-empt expected stress incontinence. *Int Urogynecol J* 2008;19:773–82.

Sermet-Gaudelus I, Bianchi ML, Garabedian M, et al. European cystic fibrosis bone mineralisation guidelines. *J Cyst Fibros* 2011;10:S16–23.

Shead EL, Haworth CS, Gunn E, et al. Osteoclastogenesis during infective exacerbations in patients with cystic fibrosis. *Am J Resp Crit Care Med* 2006;174:306–11.

Tangprichu V, Kelly V Stephenson A, et al. An Update on the Screening, Diagnosis, Management, and Treatment of Vitamin D Deficiency in Individuals with Cystic Fibrosis: Evidence-based recommendations from the Cystic Fibrosis Foundation. *J Clin Endocrinol Metab*;2012, 97:1082–93.

Thornton J, Rangaraj S. Disease modifying anti-rheumatic drugs in people with cystic fibrosis-related arthritis. *Cochrane Database Syst Rev* 2012 Sep12;9:CD007336.

Chapter 10

Psychological aspects of CF care

Alistair JA Duff and Helen Oxley

Key points

- Psychological assessment and support is essential post-diagnosis, whether in infancy or later

- Behavioural difficulties are common in pre-school children. Mealtime behaviours can be particularly problematic but children respond well to joint nutritional and psychological intervention

- Adherence remains a significant psychosocial challenge. There is growing evidence for the effectiveness of psychological techniques and therapies for improving this

- Transition to adult CF services is a process which should begin in early adolescence and involve the entire CF team

- Surveillance for emotional problems in children and their carers and adults is important. A significant minority of CF patients experience anxiety, depression, or other emotional difficulties. Good access to specialist psychosocial services within CF teams is essential. Other members of the MDT also require psychological skills to support patients and families

- Lung transplantation can prolong life with quality for those with end-stage disease; however, the psychosocial impact can be considerable

- Palliative care skills are a core competency for adult CF team-members

10.1 Introduction

Living with CF can be psychosocially demanding for patients and their relatives. The condition and its management affect people's ability to respond to everyday tasks and unique life events. Mutation class-specific therapies have established a new era of CF care and have given patients and their families renewed hope.

Current care has led to increasing median survival rates, but this has been achieved at the cost of a corresponding increase in the burden of treatment which individuals find arduous, time-consuming, and intrusive. Most children leaving paediatric care are well enough to take up the full opportunities of young adulthood with a good quality of life (QoL).

Adults with CF, some of whom have lived for years beyond their own expectation, now form the majority of the UK CF population. Many have jobs or are in further education and some have families of their own. However, CF still leads to respiratory failure and patients continue to face the possibility of prolonged periods of ill-health and reduced QoL before death.

This chapter considers the key psychosocial challenges in contemporary clinical CF care.

10.2 **Diagnosis**

Psychological support following diagnosis is vital. As a result of newborn screening, this now commonly occurs during infancy although can still take place in adulthood.

Whatever the age at diagnosis, helping patients, parents, and relatives adapt psychologically is crucial. This involves a combination of education and counselling.

10.2.1 **Education**

Parents need to learn about what life is going to be like with a child growing up with CF, ensuring balance between managing a complex health condition and enabling their child to grow with good self-esteem.

Clinicians must motivate and support as well as educate. Early information invariably focuses on CF and management, but 'flow' must be individualized and ought to be interactive. Educators must remember that memory is the residue of thought, and engaging people in an 'exchange of information' is essential, whereby what they think about a topic is elicited before new information is presented. This should be followed by questioning about their new understanding. The process is highly effective in increasing knowledge retention (see Figure 10.1)

- Elicit; what is already known
- Provide; new information/facts
- Elicit; new understanding

Individuals, particularly those under stress, remember only part of the consultations they attend. Teams also need to:

- Summarize key facts
- Provide written treatment plans
- Recommend reliable web-based support (see Appendix for Internet-based resources)

10.2.2 **Early intervention**

Programmes typically offer parents a combination of teaching and support, delivered to individuals, couples, or groups. Common parental emotional reactions to diagnosis include:

- Anxiety and/or depressive symptoms
- Grief reactions or chronic sorrow
- Relationship difficulties and role re-evaluation
- Increased family strain and struggling to balance the needs of the child with CF and the rest of the family

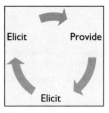

Figure 10.1 The Elicit–Provide–Elicit cycle

Although some parents become overwhelmed, many do not and they can integrate CF care into their child's daily routines, gain knowledge and skills, and adhere to the complex daily regimen. Contact with a CF psychologist is desirable at some stage post diagnosis.

Many parents want contact with other parents. Holding regular parent support groups must be considered and actively facilitated. These can address both emotional and practical aspects of raising a child with CF. Systematic review has shown that parents, especially mothers, have increased psychological problems (Berge and Patterson, 2004), particularly anxiety (which almost certainly relates to attending clinic, waiting for growth and spirometry results, and identification of new bacterial growth).

10.3 **Childhood**

For many young people with CF, childhood can be a time of comparative freedom from persistent exacerbation and treatment. However, parents often worry about how CF and treatment affects their child, particularly when behavioural problems threaten to undermine care.

Like all parents, those whose child has CF need to establish good routines and deal with oppositional behaviours. These are so common in pre-school children that they are known as the 'terrible twos'. It is important that such behaviours do not become entrenched and impinge on cooperation with treatment and procedures.

10.3.1 **Feeding behaviour problems**

Mealtime behaviour problems are one of the most frequently cited difficulties in pre-school children with CF. These can comprise:

- Lack of appetite
- Food refusal
- Restricted food choices
- Leaving the table during mealtimes
- Crying

These can lead to parental anxiety over calorie intake and to parental responses including, for example, coaxing, force-feeding, and setting different meals. In turn, these responses unintentionally 'reinforce' the unwanted feeding behaviours. As nutrition and growth are a significant part of CF management, it is important that parents receive timely support and guidance.

Dietetic assessment can be augmented with feeding behaviour scales (e.g. the Behavioral Pediatric Feeding Assessment Scale, BPFAS) to identify problems early. Effective dietetic guidance for parents includes:

- Having meals as a family together
- Keeping mealtimes to no more than 20 minutes
- Giving smaller portions and reward success (i.e. an empty plate)
- If necessary, having more frequent, smaller mealtimes
- Avoiding coaxing, bribery, and force-feeding
- Not making alternative meals

If problems persist, then joint nutritional and psychological intervention has been shown to be effective in improving oral intake and growth.

10.3.2 **Procedural distress**

Children of all ages find venepuncture one of the most frightening aspects of hospital visits. This can result in such fear and distress that the child attempts to avoid procedures, ultimately leading to sedation or restraint (or both). Young children with CF are also known to struggle with cough swabs and sputum sampling. They typically undergo many such procedures during routine care and it is important that they learn to cope with these, if longer-term 'phobic' levels of fear and compromised care are to be avoided.

Psychological interventions are known to be effective and form the basis of several guidelines. The challenge is integrating these into routine practice, the essentials of which are outlined in Table 10.1 and reviewed by Duff and colleagues (2012).

10.3.3 **Emotional difficulties**

Like all children, those with CF face key psychosocial developmental tasks of developing self-esteem, confidence, and independence. CF can interrupt these tasks, particularly when children and young people 'feel different' from their peers.

Emotional problems include: anhedonia (inability to gain pleasure from enjoyable experiences), social withdrawal, sleep disturbance, worries over treatment or friendships, and physical problems made worse by worry. In some circumstances, if prolonged, these can lead to clinical episodes of depression and anxiety for which there are well-established treatment protocols.

Nonetheless, there remains a significant minority of patients in whom symptoms can go undiagnosed and this warrants routine surveillance (using either psychometrics or interview or both).

Starting high school is a time where children with CF are potentially emotionally vulnerable and every opportunity to increase confidence and independence should be taken, making every contact count.

Table 10.1 The 6 'Ps'	
Prior Knowledge	What is the child's experience of 'needles'?
	What coping strategies have worked well?
	Are there any technical/access difficulties?
	If child is highly fearful, mark this in the notes
	Avoid inexperienced practitioners attempting venepuncture
Preparation	Prepare equipment in advance
	Undertake the procedure as soon as possible in the 'consultation'
	Give children information on anticipated sensations
	Rehearse the procedure
	Actively encourage parents to stay
Pharmacology	Consider topical anaesthetic options
	Use conscious sedation if necessary
Participation	Involve the child. Let them remove plasters, and choose and clean the site,
	Ask if they want to watch or not
	Give parents explicit instructions
Permission to make a noise	Tell children 'it's OK to scream or cry'
	Avoid telling them to 'be brave'
Patience	Give children the option to halt the procedure if they become frightened
	Take a break
	Re-introduce the procedure step-by-step

10.4 Adolescence

In terms of psychological development, teenagers need to achieve a sense of self-identity and independence from their parents, develop physical and intellectual maturity and form relationships outside their family. Taking on these challenges, when psychosocial abilities are maturing, can negatively affect attempts to assume responsibility for CF care.

Teams need to actively help families navigate from parent-guided to self-guided care by adopting adolescent-friendly approaches in clinics and wards, and by gradually increasing teenagers' participation in consultations and treatment decision-making. This sets a healthy context within which to address any adherence problems which typically emerge during this phase. (Adherence to treatments is addressed in section 10.7).

Encouragingly, the evidence is that this group are psychologically well-adapted and well-functioning with good QoL. Estimated rates of moderate/severe depression are low in adolescents with CF in the UK, although anxiety has been shown to be higher.

10.5 Transition to adult services

The importance of effective preparation and planned transfer to adult CF services is well-recognized. Transition to adulthood is not an event but a process that begins in early adolescence and involves close interdisciplinary working in both paediatric and adult teams (see Table 10.2 and Chapter 2).

Barriers to effective transition

- Patients who are sick or who deteriorate rapidly
- Fears about adult care or the transfer process (e.g. perceptions of 'moving closer to death' or increased risk of cross-infection)
- Low self-esteem or self-efficacy

Table 10.2 Psychosocial benchmarks for effective transition	
Paediatric team	• Begin preparation for transition during early adolescence by encouraging appropriate levels of self-care, self-advocacy, and participation in decision-making • Reinforce positive messages about contemporary adult life with CF • Address any errant heath beliefs (e.g. 'some exposure to infection is good for immunity') • Review progress annually and link treatment goals with life goals • Help parents anticipate their own changing roles • Reassure parents that they will not be 'excluded' by the adult CF team if the patient wishes them to be involved • Make detailed preparation for transfer on an individual transition plan, led by a key worker who has close familial involvement
Paediatric and adult teams	• Arrange meetings with adult CF team and visits to the adult centre • Use 'readiness' as an indicator of transfer rather than 'age' (up to the age limit of the paediatric service). Widely regarded tools to prepare and assess readiness are available (e.g. 'Ready Steady Go; see Appendix) • Assess and document barriers to transfer and address these • Ensure effective communication (both verbal and written) between teams and share detailed information at transfer
Adult team	• Quickly establish appropriate care plans and goals based on transition information and developmental needs • Regularly update knowledge of adolescent and young adult psychosocial development

10.6 **Psychological difficulties in adulthood**

Adults with CF have to deal with many stressors leading to some developing psychological problems that require specialist intervention. At times, many have difficulty in coping, lowering their QoL as a result. Those diagnosed with CF in adulthood have may have a range of emotional reactions, including shock, feelings of confusion, and increased awareness of death, and need specially tailored education about CF to meet their needs for information most appropriately (Widerman, 2003).

10.6.1 **Identifying specific psychological difficulties**

Early identification of adult patients at 'high risk' of psychological difficulties and timely referral to the CF psychologist is important. CF teams need to be aware of early signs of emerging psychological problems and of the potential risks of deteriorating psychological health for people with CF. Specialist psychological surveillance should form part of the annual assessment for adults with CF. Psychometric scales can help identify some problems quickly but recognition of others may need more specific questioning as part of 'face-to-face' assessment.

10.6.2 **Psychopathology**

Adulthood can bring many challenges for people with CF, including new diagnoses/medical complications, traumatic medical events, high treatment burden, and the need to make difficult decisions (e.g. about work and family life). Wide-ranging psychological issues can arise for adults (see Box 10.1) which can impact negatively on treatment adherence and QoL. A significant minority of patients report having moderate/severe disordered mood and preventing and treating significant psychological difficulties should be a key goal for teams (i.e. through specialist early intervention and maximizing coping strategies).

10.6.3 **Pain**

Recent review has concluded that there is a high incidence of pain amongst CF patients (chest and abdominal pain being the most commonly reported). Pain was negatively associated with pulmonary exacerbations, QoL, and adherence. With around half of all patients under-reporting pain, there is a real need for more proactive assessment during routine

---

Box 10.1 Psychological issues for adults with CF

- Anxiety disorders (including panic attacks, phobias, generalized anxiety disorder, and obsessive–compulsive disorder)
- Depression or significant low mood (which can involve self-harm and suicidal ideation or acts), anhedonia, and demoralization
- Post-traumatic stress reactions to medical events (e.g. haemoptysis, pneumothorax)
- Low self-esteem and confidence
- Anger
- Sleep disturbance
- Distorted body image
- Disordered eating
- Family or relationship difficulties
- Substance misuse
- Problems managing CF (including coping with increasingly invasive procedures and deteriorating health)

clinic visits, with robust plans being put in place for management, including psychological interventions (Havermans et al., 2013).

10.6.4 Psychological interventions

The entire CF team has a role in providing psychological care and support for adults with CF. Teams need to work collaboratively with patients who are usually well-informed about their condition, and who often expect to be involved in treatment decisions. Some members of the team also need additional skills to provide emotional support to patients at difficult times. CF specialist social workers may undertake this role, as well as providing advice on benefits, higher education and employment issues, housing, and accessing community-based resources as required.

CF psychologists can support the psychological care provided by the rest of the team through training and consultation, and can also deliver specialized psychological interventions for a wide range of psychological issues, health management issues, and mental health problems.

Whilst the effectiveness of different psychological interventions in CF specifically has not been investigated in detail, the evidence base for cognitive behaviour therapy (CBT) is strong for many psychological problems and must be made available in the CF team. Other widely used and potentially helpful psychological interventions include: motivational interviewing, systemic therapies, solution-focused approaches, and 'mindfulness' techniques. Support for families of patients is also essential and may be provided by the CF social worker, alongside their other responsibilities.

10.7 Adherence to treatment

Good adherence is taking treatment in the right way at the right time. It is strongly associated with better health outcomes and a reduced risk of hospitalization. In contrast, sub-optimal adherence is linked to treatment failure, lower QoL, reduced baseline lung functioning and higher morbidity, and is predictive of intravenous antibiotic requirements. Improving adherence has become one of the most important psychosocial challenges in CF care.

Treatments that are time-consuming, afford no immediate benefit or are intrusive are least likely to be adhered to. In CF these are physiotherapy, dietary recommendations, and the use of nebulizers. The latter gives particular cause for concern with their prominence in respiratory drug delivery.

There are 5 general principles that CF teams need to establish to facilitate optimal adherence amongst patients:

1. Accept that partial adherence is normal
2. Establish an empathic team approach
3. Avoid blame or criticism
4. Provide written copies of treatment plans
5. Prioritise and simplify regimes, setting realistic goals

Improving adherence often requires the combination of several approaches; organizational, educational, motivational, and behavioural (see Table 10.3). Psychological techniques have more chance of success if they are embedded in a strong team culture of openness and honesty. Team members actively listening to patients and engaging them in their healthcare is the vital first step; eliciting their health beliefs about medicines or therapies is the second. A useful conceptual framework is to view these as 'necessities' or 'concerns'. Those with more 'concern-based' beliefs are more likely to have poorer adherence.

Table 10.3 Methods to improve adherence	
Approach	**Exemplar**
Organizational • Shared team approach • Increase accessibility • Patient-friendly approach	• Develop common principles • Outreach clinics, telephone support • Simplify treatments, adapt treatments to lifestyles
Provide education • CF, treatment, side-effects • Adherence problems in complex regimens • Barriers to adherence • Improving adherence • Relapse prevention	**How**—Leaflets, videos, mobile 'apps', slide-shows, handouts, demonstrations **Where**—During routine clinic visits, home-visits, telephone consultations **By whom**—Entire CF team
Motivational • Express empathy • Respect choice to 'change or not' • Identify discrepancies between beliefs, behaviours, and goals • Clarify treatment goals and remove barriers to change • Work *with* resistance • Provide regular feedback • Support the development of patient self-efficacy	• Listen to and understand patients' perspectives • Consider advantages/disadvantages of change (avoid arguing *for* change) • Accept that goals of treatment vary • Never directly confront patients • Positively reinforce any small changes or contemplation of change • Develop patients' growing sense that they *can* achieve change
Behavioural • Self-monitoring • Set achievable goals • Behavioural contracting • Positive feedback and reinforcement	• Patient diaries • Write 'contracts' with patients about specific adherence behaviours required • Systematically encourage and reward

Behavioural approaches to adherence depend on patients' readiness to change. Perceptual (or emotional) barriers are often present in those unwilling to openly recognize adherence problems or who lack motivation to change. The effectiveness of addressing these issues within the context of a motivational interviewing framework is gaining in both empirical and clinical strength.

There is emerging proof that CF-specific training in motivational interviewing has lasting learning outcomes and changes clinical practice.

10.8 **Quality of life (QoL)**

Measuring health-related QoL yields important information about the subjective impact of CF upon patients' lives. Patient-reported outcomes are an essential part of the evaluation of therapies and interventions and are as important for children, young people, and their families as they are for adults.

There are several health QoL measures but only a few specifically for use with CF patients and families. One that is used internationally is the Cystic Fibrosis Questionnaire (CFQ), which has 12 domains including physical functioning, emotional state, social limitations, body image, and treatment constraints. Language and country-specific versions are available (e.g. the CFQ-UK).

> **Box 10.2 Key psychological tasks in end-of-life care**
>
> - Help teams carry out advance care planning with patients, who can then make informed choices and communicate these
> - Ensure that patients' psychological, spiritual, and existential needs are listened to and addressed
> - Identify barriers to optimal palliative care
> - Deliver psychological interventions for depression, anxiety, anticipatory grief, pain, and insomnia
> - Discuss bereavement issues with families (and fellow patients)
> - Facilitate peer support for team members
> - Assist in ensuring that necessary palliative care training is met

10.9 **Transplantation and end-of-life care**

Deaths occurring at comparatively young ages, after long relationships between patients, families, and teams, and where prognosis can be hard to predict, can make end-stage care in CF particularly complex and distressing.

10.9.1 **Transplantation**

For patients with end-stage disease, lung transplantation may be considered for those without absolute contra-indications. This now usually occurs in the adult CF population, although still occasionally in paediatrics.

The process of referral for transplantation, assessment, and living with declining health whilst on a waiting list is psychologically stressful. Being told of the need for transplant referral and making a decision about active listing may necessitate additional psychological support.

Assessment of psychosocial factors, such as psychological problems, lack of social support that could impact upon transplant outcome, and issues with adherence to treatment, are all important to the transplant assessment. These require close communication between CF and transplant centres.

10.9.2 **Palliative care**

The goal of 'a good death' is more likely to be achieved if CF teams have the skills to address these difficult issues without avoidance. The possibility of transplantation can complicate end-of-life planning, and CF patients may demonstrate oscillation between desire for information and avoidance of this. However, talking about end-of-life care and advanced planning gives patients opportunities to make well-informed decisions and choices, and to consider what they have achieved in their lives and what they have left to do before they die (see Box 10.2).

Using the principles of palliative care is important, even if these need adapting for CF care. It gives teams opportunities to consider often under-diagnosed symptoms (e.g. pain and nausea), and to ameliorate psychological distress.

References

Berge JM, Patterson JM. Cystic fibrosis and the family: a review and critique of the literature. *Families, Systems & Health* 2004; 22:74–100.

Braithwaite M, Philip J, Tranberg H, et al. End of life care in CF: patients, families and staff experiences and unmet needs. *J Cyst Fibrosis* 2011;10:253–7.

Duff AJA, Gaskell SL, Jacobs K, et al. Management of distressing procedures in children and young people: time to adhere to the guidelines. *Arch Dis Child* 2012;97:1–4.

Havermans T, Kolpeart K, De Boeck K, et al. Pain in CF: Review of the literature. *J Cyst Fibrosis* 2013;12:423–30.

Kettler LJ, Sawyer SM, Winefied HR, et al. Determinants of adherence in adults with cystic fibrosis. *Thorax* 2002;5:459–64.

Stark LJ, Quittner AL, Powers SW, et al. A randomized clinical trial of behavioural intervention and nutrition education to improve caloric intake and weight in children with cystic fibrosis. *Arch Pediatr Adolesc Med* 2009;163:915–21.

Widerman E. Knowledge, interests and educational needs of adults receiving a cystic fibrosis diagnosis after age 18. *J Cyst Fibrosis* 2003;2:97–104.

Chapter 11

Lung transplantation

John Blaikley and Andrew J Fisher

Key points

- Lung transplantation should be considered a treatment option for severe CF lung disease uncontrolled on maximal medical therapy
- Lung transplantation is not a cure for CF and ongoing CF team care should continue after lung transplantation
- Referral to the transplant centre should be made in a timely fashion using international referral criteria as a guide
- Pre-transplant assessment of physical, functional, microbiological, and psychological parameters is used to determine candidate suitability
- Pre-transplant optimization of physical functioning and nutrition is essential to increase the chance of a successful transplant outcome
- Immunosuppressive drugs are required lifelong after lung transplant and are associated with significant side effects which can themselves cause morbidity
- Early complications include primary graft dysfunction, infection, and acute rejection of the transplanted lungs
- Long-term survival is limited by development of chronic graft dysfunction termed chronic lung allograft dysfunction (CLAD)

11.1 Introduction

Lung transplantation, when successful, offers the possibility of an active and extended life to selected patients with severe end-stage lung disease that is failing on maximal medical therapy.

The modern era of lung transplant started in the early 1980s. Currently around 4000 lung transplants are performed each year worldwide. Advances in patient selection, surgical techniques, antibiotic and immunosuppressive medication regimens have steadily improved outcomes with many lung transplant recipients able to survive in excess of 10 years.

The primary aim of lung transplantation is to improve survival with the secondary benefit of improving quality of life. Due to the shortage of donor organs, lung transplantation will rarely be performed for improvement in quality of life alone. As a result, indicators of disease severity and of an adverse prognosis without transplantation must also be satisfied in potential candidates.

Due to the limited supply of donor organs, each patient referred must be assessed for suitability and the likelihood of a successful outcome determined before being placed on the active lung transplant waiting list.

11.2 **Lung transplantation for CF**

Due to advances in the organization of CF care and increasingly prompt and aggressive treatment of infections, people with CF are surviving longer with an average survival age of >40 years.

CF is the third most common condition for which lung transplantation is performed, accounting for 16% of all lung transplants worldwide.

Post-transplant survival for CF is among the highest of all transplantable chronic lung conditions with an 83% 1-year survival rate, 69% 3-year survival, and 60% 5-year survival worldwide (*International Society of Heart and Lung Transplant* registry data). However, centres very experienced in performing lung transplants for CF can exceed this, with some achieving a median survival of over 10 years.

Lung disease is the primary cause of death in >80% of CF patients meaning that lung transplantation is a treatment option required by many. Despite attempts to increase organ donation, demand still significantly outstrips supply, waiting lists are growing, and there remains a significant number of deaths among those on the waiting list.

11.2.1 **Surgical approach**

All CF patients require a bilateral lung transplant to minimize the risk of re-infection due to chronic bacterial and fungal colonization from the colonized native lung.

Bilateral lung transplantation is often performed through a 'clamshell' or transverse incision (see Figure 11.1). The native lungs are removed, usually with the patient on cardiopulmonary bypass or extracorporeal membrane oxygenation (ECMO), and the new lungs implanted one at a time (often referred to as a single, sequential lung transplant).

11.2.2 **When to refer**

Each patient has a window of opportunity when the benefits of transplantation, with regards to survival and quality of life, outweigh the risks of surgery and peri-operative complications.

Patients should be referred early enough to prevent them becoming too sick for transplantation if their condition deteriorates. Furthermore, timely referral is paramount due to the shortage of donor organs and the risk of death on the waiting list.

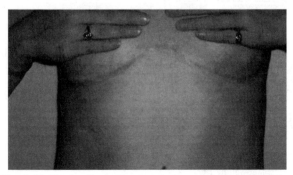

Figure 11.1 Clamshell incision on a female CF patient who has previously undergone bilateral lung transplantation.

Once listed for lung transplant, the waiting time can vary widely depending on blood group, size, and the condition of other candidates on the waiting list. Current opinion is that a patient should be referred when their predicted 2-year survival is approximately 50%. This can be difficult to ascertain due to the heterogeneous nature of CF lung disease and the absence of an accurate prognostic model for CF lung disease, therefore international guidelines for assessment (Box 11.1) have been published.

Most transplant centres would prefer early referral to ensure enough time for rational assessment of the patient, management of any areas of concern, optimization of the patient's pre-transplant condition, and ultimately patient education to allow an unhurried and informed decision regarding lung transplantation.

11.2.3 Recipient selection

Lung transplantation carries a significant morbidity and mortality risk. To ensure the best possible outcome, patients are assessed using strict selection criteria (Box 11.2 and Box 11.3) and their pre-transplant condition is optimized as best possible.

Conditions or targets, such as weight management or physical conditioning, may be set by the transplant centre which must be achieved before transplantation is considered appropriate.

Box 11.1 CF-specific referral criteria (ISHLT guidelines)*

- FEV_1 <30% predicted or rapid decline in FEV_1 (especially if female and <18 years)
- Increasing frequency of exacerbations requiring intravenous antibiotics
- Exacerbation of pulmonary disease requiring ITU stay
- Refractory or recurrent pneumothoraces
- Recurrent haemoptysis not controlled by embolization

Regardless of the above criteria, imminent referral should be considered in the context of:
- Oxygen dependent respiratory failure
- Hypercapnia
- Pulmonary hypertension

* ISHLT: International Society of Heart and Lung Transplantation

---

Box 11.2 Absolute contra-indications to lung transplantation

- Malignancy in last 2 years (excluding BCC and SCC of skin)
- Untreatable advanced dysfunction of additional major organ system (unless a multi-organ transplant is being considered)
- Documented ongoing non-compliance
- Untreatable psychiatric or psychological condition affecting ability to cooperate or comply with treatment
- Absence of reliable, consistent, social support system
- Current substance addiction or excessive alcohol use
- Known immunosuppression drug intolerance
- Current smoker
- Inability to adequately treat pulmonary infections*
- Colonization with *Burkholderia cepacia genomovar* III (most centres worldwide)*

* CF-specific contra-indications

> Box 11.3 Relative contra-indications to lung transplantation
>
> - Age >65 years (single lung) or >60 years (bilateral lung)
> - Critical or unstable condition
> - Severely limited functional status with poor rehabilitation potential
> - Colonization with highly resistant or highly virulent organisms
> - Severe or symptomatic osteoporosis
> - Invasive mechanical ventilation
> - Comorbidities (no end-organ damage, must be optimally treated)
> - Poorly controlled extra-pulmonary CF-disease manifestations*
> - Poor nutritional status: BMI<18 *
> - Liver cirrhosis with hepatic dysfunction and uncontrolled portal hypertension (potential for lung/liver transplant in selected candidates and centres)*
> - Colonization with *Mycobacterium abscessus**
> - Intra-cavitary Aspergillus situated near the pleura*
> - Severe pleural thickening*
> - Malignancy in last 5 years
> - Acute extra-pulmonary sepsis/uncontrolled systemic infection
> - Significant chest wall or spinal deformity
> * Contra-indications specific to CF

11.2.4 **Special considerations in CF**

Lung transplantation will improve respiratory disease, but extra-pulmonary disease in the sinuses, intestines, pancreas, and upper airways remains and can influence outcome post transplantation.

Sinus and upper airways disease

Colonization of the sinuses, upper respiratory tract, and large airways with multi-resistant organisms are a potential risk for pulmonary re-infection post-transplantation. Although isolation of pre-transplant organisms after transplantation is common, there is no evidence that sinus surgery and washout pre-transplant affects outcomes post-transplantation. Many transplant centres use nebulized antibiotics in an attempt to prevent clinical infection in the context of immunosuppression.

Pneumothoraces

Management of recurrent pneumothoraces can present problems in the management of patients awaiting lung transplant. Current recommendations are to perform the minimum intervention required to control and stabilize the patient's condition. Studies suggest that patients who have undergone previous pleural procedures do not have adverse outcomes after lung transplant compared to those who did not. Blood pleurodesis has not been shown to offer any benefit over other interventions.

Respiratory Infections

Improvements in peri-operative mortality in the CF population may be due to advances in microbiological testing and the use of targeted antibiotic regimes at the time of transplant.

CF patients are often chronically infected with multi- or pan-resistant organisms and the risk of seeding infections to the pleura, or systemically, at the time of transplantation, are

> **Box 11.4** Organisms not associated with an increase in mortality
>
> - Multi-drug *Pseudomonas aeruginosa*
> - *Staphylococcus aureus*
> - Methicillin-resistant *Staphylococcus aureus*
> - *Stenotrophomonas maltophilia*
> - *Alcaligenes xylosoxidans*
> - *Aspergillus fumigatus*
> - Atypical mycobacterium (excluding *Mycobacterium abscessus*)

considerable. Repeated antibiotic use can lead to multiple antibiotic hypersensitivities in this population, limiting the antibiotics available for use. Desensitization may need to occur pre-transplant if there are limited antibiotic options (see Chapter 14).

To reduce peri-operative infection risks to an acceptable level an antibiotic regimen must be found that adequately treats recipient organisms before transplant can be considered. Patients may not be listed for transplant until an effective combination of antibiotics can be identified.

Some centres use multiple combination synergy testing to find the best combination of antibiotics for use at the time of transplant. It is important to update the transplant centre regularly about recent infections and antibiotic use, in addition to sending regular sputum samples, as this can affect the antibiotics used during the post-operative period.

Many organisms initially thought to affect transplant outcomes adversely have not been proven to increase mortality in isolation (Box 11.4). The risk that specific infections contribute depends on the presence of other relative contra-indications.

- Only one study has suggested that multi-drug or pan-resistant *Pseudomonas aeruginosa* increases mortality post transplantation. Two other studies have shown that pan-resistant organisms had no effect on mortality. Pan-resistant *pseudomonas* is therefore not an absolute contra-indication to transplantation

- Intracavitary *Aspergillus fumigatus* or mycetoma situated near the pleura can be seeded at the time of transplant. Aggressive and comprehensive treatment is needed, but such patients have been successfully transplanted

- Atypical mycobacteria other than *Mycobacterium abscessus* are not a contra-indication to transplantation as long as they have been adequately controlled

Some organisms have been associated with an increased morbidity and mortality in some centres after lung transplantation:

- *Mycobacterium abscessus,* a rapidly growing mycobacterium, has a high risk of recurrence since it is extremely difficult to eradicate and often infects soft tissues. Removal of the lungs does not necessarily indicate complete removal of the organism. It is associated with significantly increased morbidity and mortality and requires assessment on an individual patient basis to assess risk

- *Burkholderia cenocepacia* has been shown to be detrimental to survival post transplantation with a 30–40% increase in mortality (50% survival at 1 year). This degree of increased mortality acts as a contra-indication to lung transplantation in most centres worldwide. Other organisms within the *Burkholderia cepacia* complex do not carry this increased risk in well-selected recipients

11.2.5 **Non-pulmonary manifestations of CF and lung transplantation**

Non-pulmonary manifestations of CF can have a major impact in the early post-operative period.

Pancreatic insufficiency

More than 85% of patients with CF require pancreatic enzyme supplementation due to pancreatic insufficiency. Pancreatic enzymes should be given with ciclosporin to improve absorption, as adequate levels of immunosuppressant can be difficult to achieve in CF patients.

Distal intestinal obstruction syndrome (DIOS)

Gastrointestinal complications such as abdominal pain and diarrhoea are common after lung transplantation in patients with CF. DIOS is the most significant early GI complication with a frequency of approximately 20%. Active prevention is vital, with early administration of pancreatic enzymes and vigilance to enable early diagnosis and prompt treatment (see Chapter 7).

Gastro oesophageal reflux disease (GORD)

GORD is common in CF patients and can worsen after surgery due to gastro paresis and potential damage to the vagus nerve. Reflux is associated with development of chronic lung allograft dysfunction and so needs to be treated promptly and aggressively, with fundoplication if necessary.

Liver disease

Liver disease occurs in one-quarter of patients with CF and is a major complication that is becoming more relevant as extra-hepatic disease is more effectively treated. Patients with advanced liver disease undergoing lung transplantation have a high morbidity and mortality resulting from post-operative hepatic insufficiency. A combined liver–lung transplant may be considered for those patients with end-stage pulmonary disease and progressive advanced liver disease.

Nutrition

Most transplant centres will not consider transplantation if BMI is <18, as poor nutrition is associated with poor outcomes post transplantation. Often overnight nasogastric tube feeding or placement of a percutaneous gastrostomy tube is recommended to maintain a safe weight (see Chapter 7). A minimum weight may be stipulated at assessment, and even once listed the patient may not be transplanted if below this target weight.

Diabetes mellitus

CF-related diabetes occurs in 30% of adult patients. Good glycaemic control is important as uncontrolled diabetes can adversely affect outcomes such as surgical healing and prolonged infection in the post-operative period (see Chapter 8). Good control of CF-related diabetes helps to maintain weight in the pre-transplant period. 20% of patients develop diabetes after transplantation due to a combination of calcineurin inhibitors and high-dose steroids, with a particularly strong tendency to this amongst the CF population.

Osteoporosis

Osteopenia is common in the CF population and should be considered for treatment with bisphosphonates with calcium and vitamin D supplementation before transplantation (see

Chapter 9). Bone mineral density will be further reduced post transplantation by the use of steroid and immunosuppressants.

Renal dysfunction

Renal dysfunction may also occur in the CF population as a result of aminoglycoside use or diabetes. After transplantation, the immunosuppressant regimen can produce renal damage and 20% of lung transplant recipients require renal replacement therapy either temporarily or permanently. A key part of the evaluation process is therefore to assess renal function. Every effort should be made to preserve renal function both before and after transplantation ensuring that this complication is minimized.

Other considerations

Mechanical ventilation is considered a relative contra-indication to transplantation in most transplant centres. In the general population, invasive ventilation is a risk factor for post-transplant mortality but some studies suggest this is not the case in CF. There is no consensus between transplant centres but if the patient has been assessed and listed before intubation and there is a short ventilation time, they may be successfully transplanted (see section 11.3.3).

Chronic *Clostridium difficile* carriage occurs in many CF patients and can cause infection in the early post-transplant period due to aggressive use of antibiotics and immunosuppression. Presentation is often atypical, with an absence of diarrhoea. Complications include toxic megacolon and fibrosing colonopathy, which frequently requires surgery and is associated with a high mortality.

11.3 **The process of lung transplantation**

11.3.1 **Pre-transplant**

Patients will undergo a 3–5 day assessment process with numerous investigations performed to assess disease severity and suitability for transplant. These will also highlight areas for medical optimisation and investigate the patient's ability to cope psychologically with transplantation issues.

Transplantation is a major life event and constitutes a substantial emotional, financial, and physical ordeal for the candidate and their carers. For this reason, it is essential that a robust support system exists to be able to stay with the candidate at the hospital at the time of transplant and provide support during the peri-operative recovery period.

The patient is committing to a lifetime of immunosuppressive medication and susceptibility to infection. Compliance with medication, minimizing infection risk, following post-transplant management advice and lifestyle advice is essential for a successful outcome.

To minimize organ ischaemic time, patients are often notified to come to the transplant centre whilst the potential donor lungs are still being assessed. This might lead to the potential transplant being cancelled. This can happen a number of times before a candidate is successfully transplanted.

11.3.2 **Recipient and donor matching**

Matching of a recipient to donor organs is done by blood group and predicted total lung capacity (TLC) using height, age, and sex. Race and gender have no bearing on matching.

Predicted recipient TLC is matched to predicted donor TLC to match for size. The severity of illness is considered, but time on the list is not a prioritization indicator for transplantation.

Increasingly it is recognized that donor-specific antibodies are an important determinant of survival post-transplant. Virtual cross-match is when the tissue typing of the donor is matched against the preformed antibody profile of the potential recipient on paper (i.e. virtual) rather than in the lab. If the donor possesses a particular HLA that the recipient has antibodies against, then the virtual cross-match is positive and many centres will not transplant. More recently, centres are stratifying the antibody titre in the recipient and if antibody levels are low will transplant against a positive virtual cross-match. It is important, however, to minimize blood transfusions, which can generate donor specific antibodies and thus increase the likelihood of a virtual cross-match.

As the shortage of donor organs limits who can be transplanted, patients will often be asked to consent for extended donor or EVLP (*ex-vivo* lung perfusion). Extended donor criteria are specific for each centre and describe a relaxation of the original ISHLT-ideal donor criteria. Specific examples include the acceptance of organs from smokers, donors up to the age of 65 (normally 55 years is the cut-off), or the presence of pulmonary oedema. These extended criteria organs are only accepted if they pass normal physiological measurements of acceptability. EVLP is a method of perfusing the lung *ex-vivo*, minimizing the cold ischaemic time whilst more detailed assessment is performed on marginal organs that do not meet initial acceptable physiological criteria of acceptance. Initial trials have shown that in the short term, these organs have comparable outcomes compared to those organs accepted without EVLP.

11.3.3 **ECMO and NIV as a bridge to transplantation**

An unexpected deterioration in a patient's condition can lead to ventilation, if they are listed as a transplant candidate. It is important to prevent the muscle wastage associated with endotracheal intubation as this impacts the post-operative course post transplantation. Two main options are open to the clinician; non-invasive ventilation is preferable but this has only limited ability to correct hypoxemia or type 2 respiratory failure (see Chapter 6). Extracorporeal membrane oxygenation (ECMO) may, in carefully selected candidates, act as a bridge to transplant for a few weeks. Venous blood undergoes extra-corporeal oxygenation and is returned to the venous (V–V ECMO) or arterial system (V–A ECMO). This can only be a short-term solution due to patient deconditioning or complications related to the procedure.

11.3.4 **Post-transplant complications**

Lung transplantation often produces a dramatic change for the patient (Figure 11.2); however, most patients develop some complications after transplantation. Complications post lung transplantation can be divided into early (<6 months) and late (>6 months) (see Table 11.1 and 11.2). Shared care between the transplant centre and local CF centre is encouraged to ensure continued management of non-pulmonary CF-related disease.

Acute rejection

Acute rejection is common, occurring in up to 50% patients in the first 6 months. To allow early detection and prompt treatment, some transplant centres perform regular, surveillance bronchoscopy and transbronchial biopsy during the first years after transplantation. Acute rejection is often asymptomatic or can present insidiously and non-specifically. Symptoms include low-grade fever, lethargy, and dyspnoea. When patients are being investigated, the chest X-ray can show bilateral infiltrates or small pleural effusions, and there may be a fall in pulmonary function. If acute rejection is suspected, referral to the transplant centre for consideration of transbronchial biopsy and prompt treatment with augmented immunosuppression is required.

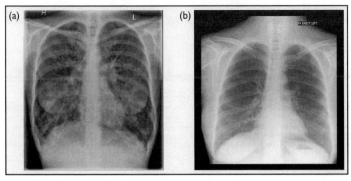

Figure 11.2 CXR of a CF patient (a) pre- and (b) post-transplantation.

Malignancy

The incidence of malignancy is increased after lung transplantation due to the effects of the immunosuppressants on immune function. Although there is an increased incidence of solid organ tumours, the commonest malignancy after transplantation is skin cancer and patients must therefore use high-factor sun-block. Cystic fibrosis patients are also at higher risk of colon cancer compared to the normal population, and therefore some centres use colonoscopy screening before and after transplantation.

Post-transplant lymphoproliferative disorder (PTLD)

PTLD is the second most common malignancy after skin cancer in solid organ transplant recipients. After lung transplantation, the incidence is 4–10%, and in the majority of cases it is driven by Epstein–Barr virus (EBV) infection. PTLD can occur in any organ including the lung, intestine, liver, and central nervous system. The most common presenting features are fever and lymphadenopathy, followed by symptoms caused by extra-nodal involvement. Asymptomatic nodules in the lung or liver can be the first sign of the condition. Diagnosis requires excisional biopsy to provide tissue for histology and evaluation of EBV status. A reduction in the level of immunosuppression (cessation of the cell cycle inhibitor) may be effective in some individuals, but those who fail to respond to this approach often require chemotherapy.

Bronchiolitis obliterans syndrome (BOS)

Long-term survival after lung transplantation is limited by the development of progressive dysfunction of the transplanted lungs, often labelled as 'chronic rejection' or chronic lung allograft dysfunction (CLAD). CLAD can be split into two different pathological entities: obliterative bronchiolitis (OB) and pulmonary fibrosis. Both entities are caused by chronic inflammation and fibrotic repair. These entities clinically are termed *Bronchiolitis obliterans* syndrome (BOS) or restrictive allograft syndrome (RAS), respectively. BOS is defined by progressive airflow obstruction in the absence of other identifiable causes of graft dysfunction. It is the most common form of CLAD, affecting 50–60% of patients surviving more than 5 years after lung transplant and has a 3-year mortality of >50%. Patients present with dyspnoea, cough, chest tightness, and a reduction in exercise capacity. The condition is often accompanied by increased bacterial infections.

Table 11.1 Early complications of lung transplantation	
Anastomotic complications	• Dehiscence
	• Stricture
	• Granulation tissue obstruction
Phrenic nerve damage	• Raised hemidiaphragm
Left recurrent laryngeal nerve damage	• Hoarse voice
Pulmonary venous thrombosis	
Primary graft dysfunction	
Venous thromboembolism	
Acute rejection	
Pulmonary infection	• Bacterial
	• Viral
	• Fungal
	• Protozoal
Non-pulmonary infection	• Mediastinitis
	• Pleural collections
Gastrointestinal	• DIOS
	• Peptic ulceration
	• GORD
	• Pseudomembraneous colitis
	• Hepatitis
CNS	• Ciclosporin related seizures
	• Multifocal leucoencephalopathy
Metabolic	• Hypo/hyperkalaemia
	• Hyponatraemia
	• Hypomagnaeseamia
	• Hypocalcaemia
	• Hypophospataemia

Onset of BOS can be insidious or acute, and its progression varies significantly and is impossible to predict initially. Possible presentations include:

- Sudden onset with rapid decline in lung function
- Insidious onset with slow, progressive decline over time
- Initial rapid decline in FEV_1 followed by a prolonged period of stability

Table 11.2 Late complications of lung transplant	
Airway complications	• Tracheo-bronchomalacia
	• Bronchial fistulae
Malignancy	• Skin
	• PTLD
	• Gastrointestinal
Chronic allograft rejection	• Obliterative bronchiolitis
Infection	• Bacterial
	• Viral
	• Fungal
	• Protozoal
Diabetes mellitus	
Hypertension	
Dyslipidaemia	
Renal Impairment	• Calcineurin inhibitor-related nephrotoxicity

A high index of suspicion, taking into account known risk factors (see Box 11.5) combined with regular surveillance of lung function by spirometry and discussion with transplant centres remain vital to early detection of BOS. BOS should be suspected in patients with an irreversible reduction in pulmonary function to <80% best post-transplant FEV_1 in whom infection and acute rejection have been excluded.

Restrictive allograft syndrome is often more rapid and severe compared to BOS. Patients present with dyspnoea associated with progressive infiltrates on the chest X-ray in the absence of any other identifiable cause. Median life expectancy is only 1 year.

11.3.5 Infections after transplantation

The risk of infection is higher after lung transplant than after other solid organ transplants. This is due to the higher immunosuppression levels required, exposure of the lung allograft to the external environment, and denervation causing impaired cough and mucociliary clearance.

Viral infections

Cytomegalovirus (CMV) is the commonest viral pathogen isolated in lung transplant recipients. CMV IgG-negative recipients in receipt of a lung from a CMV IgG-positive donor are at the highest risk of developing significant invasive disease.

The incidence of invasive disease has been significantly reduced by the use of prophylactic anti-viral strategies in CMV donor–recipient mismatches. Presentation of CMV disease can be acute, with a sudden onset of symptoms, or insidious, with low-grade temperatures, lethargy, and malaise.

CMV disease can affect any organ but most commonly affects the lung and/or the GI tract presenting with dyspnoea and/or abdominal pain and diarrhoea. Diagnosis is suspected

Box 11.5 Risk factors for CLAD

- Recurrent episodes of acute rejection
- Lymphocytic bronchitis/bronchiolitis
- *Pseudomonas* infections
- HLA mismatching
- CMV pneumonitis
- GORD
- Community-acquired respiratory virus infection
- Medical non-compliance
- Air pollution

clinically and confirmed by a significant elevation in viral DNA copies using CMV PCR or demonstration of CMV viral inclusion bodies from lung or gut biopsy.

Community-acquired respiratory viral infections are more common in lung transplant recipients and may cause acute loss of lung function. Seasonal influenza vaccination is recommended for all lung transplant recipients. Infections with such viruses have been associated with the development of chronic lung allograft dysfunction.

Bacterial infections

Bacterial infections can occur any time after lung transplantation. Infection of the transplanted lungs with *Pseudomonas* species is common in CF recipients and is often treated with regular nebulized antibiotics to reduce the risk of ongoing airway injury. Typical respiratory bacterial pathogens are more likely to be the cause of acute bacterial respiratory infections than rarer opportunistic bacteria. Mycobacterial infections, especially *Mycobacterium abscessus,* can be difficult to treat due to the antibiotic interactions with calcineurin inhibitors and the immunosuppressed state. In this scenario, close liaison is recommended with the transplant centre.

Fungal infections

Candida and *Aspergillus* species account for the vast majority of significant fungal infections. Colonization is frequent, with a combined incidence of 85%. *Aspergillus* alone is isolated in up to 45% of recipients and may be associated with bronchial anastomotic complications. It can often be detected through galactomanan, *Aspergillus* PCR, or culture. The spectrum of disease ranges from asymptomatic colonization to invasive disease and systemic fungal sepsis. Invasive aspergillosis carries a mortality of 75%.

Protozoal infections

Mortality from *Pneumocystis jirovecci* (PCP) was previously significant, but with the introduction of lifelong co-trimoxazole prophylaxis the incidence of infection has dramatically decreased.

11.4 **Immunosuppressive medication**

The majority of lung transplant recipients will receive lifelong immunosuppression using a triple-drug regime consisting of:

1. calcineurin inhibitor (ciclosporin or tacrolimus)
2. cell-cycle inhibitor (azathioprine or mycophenolate mofetil)

3. corticosteroids (prednisolone)

Important side effects include increased susceptibility to infection and calcineurin-related nephrotoxicity. Renal function needs to be carefully monitored and a degree of renal impairment is common post transplantation. Care must be taken when prescribing additional medications, especially antibiotics and anti-fungal medications due to possible interactions. Therefore, all medication should be checked for potential interactions before initiation.

11.5 Assessment of transplant recipient outside the transplant centre

Lung transplant recipients with CF may present with new symptoms to either their local district hospital or their CF centre, particularly if they live a significant distance from their transplant centre. It is important to remember that not all presentations will be related to their previous transplant. However, their status as a lung transplant recipient should always influence their management, even for common conditions.

Potential causes of acute illness can be categorized as:

1. **Transplant-specific complications**
   - acute rejection
   - rapid *bronchiolitis obliterans* syndrome
   - PTLD
   - opportunistic infections, etc.

2. **CF-specific complications**
   - CF-related liver disease
   - CF-related diabetes
   - DIOS, intussception, etc.

3. **General medical and surgical conditions**
   - pulmonary embolus
   - pneumonia
   - appendicitis, etc.

The initial approach to the sick transplant patient is the same as any other patient *except that special care should be taken before drug administration to consider potential interactions with immunosuppressive medication.*

Patient condition and onset of deterioration determines the place of care and timing of further investigations. Basic resuscitation of the critically ill patient is the same in lung transplant recipient. Full history and examination needs to be undertaken as standard.

11.5.1 Fall in lung function

If a minor fall in lung function is associated with clinical evidence of respiratory infection, then spirometry should be repeated to ensure it has normalized after treatment.

If symptoms persist, lung function fails to normalize, or there is no clinical evidence of infection, then further investigations are required.

Bronchoscopy to examine the bronchial anastomoses for strictures and bronchoalveolar lavage for culture is indicated. In addition, transbronchial biopsies are required to look for acute rejection.

Other than in exceptional circumstances, post-transplant bronchoscopy is best performed in the lung transplant centre where experienced transplant pathologists are available to report on transbronchial biopsies.

11.5.2 **Abnormal chest X-ray**

The chest X-ray appearance in a lung transplant recipient should always be checked against previous imaging as there may be chronic changes after transplant surgery.

If new infiltrates, nodules or effusions are identified and they will require further investigation. These changes are non-specific and may represent rejection, infection, or post-transplant lymphoproliferative disease. A CT scan may help to characterize the abnormalities more clearly, but invariably bronchoscopic investigations will be required.

If a nodule cannot be characterized by bronchoscopy or imaging, then a more invasive approach will be required. Early discussion with the transplant centre should take place to help guide investigations or to transfer back for further evaluation.

11.5.3 **Investigations for new-onset breathlessness**

- Chest X-ray
- Spirometry
- Flow-volume loop if available and possible
- Arterial blood gases if the oxygen saturations are low
- Sputum culture +/- nasopharyngeal lavage for viruses
- ECG

11.5.4 **Suspected infection**

If infective symptoms are present then blood cultures and a full septic screen are required as source of sepsis may be outside the lungs. Any culture samples need a full work-up for an immunocompromized host; this will need to be requested specifically from local microbiology laboratories.

Targeted antibiotics, if required, are preferable to broad-spectrum in lung transplant recipients, but clinical judgement will dictate as to whether antibiotics are required immediately. Neutropenia is not normally present in patients on immunosuppression and therefore recipients should not automatically receive neutropenic antibiotic regimes if they present with features of infection. For all transplant patients, the relevant lung transplant centre should be involved early for advice regarding management of the immunosuppression regimen as well as suitable antibiotic regimes. Prescription of the macrolide antibiotics, erythromycin and clarithromycin, are contra-indicated in patients on calcineurin inhibitors due to the risk of nephrotoxicity. In contrast, azithromycin is often used for treatment of chronic rejection rather than its antimicrobial effect.

References

Corris PA. Lung Transplantation for CF. *Curr Opin Organ Transplant* 2008;13(5):484–8.

Cypel M, Yeung JC, Liu M, et al. Normothermic ex vivo lung perfusion in clinical lung transplantation. *N Eng J Med* 2011;364(15):1431–40.

International Society of Heart and Lung Transplantation <http://www.ishlt.org>

Hadjiliadis D. Special Considerations for Patients With CF Undergoing Lung Transplantation. *Chest* 2007;131;1224–31.

Javidfar J, Bacchetta M. Bridge to lung transplantation with extracorporeal membrane oxygenation support. *Curr Opin Organ Transplant* 2012 Oct;17(5):496–502.

Liou TG, Woo MS, Cahill BC. Lung Transplantation for CF *Current Opinion in Pulmonary Medicine* 2006:12;459–63.

Lyu DM, Zamora MR. Medical complications of Lung Transplantation *Proc Am Thorac Soc* 2009:6;101–7.

Parker A, Bowles K, Bradley JA, et al. Diagnosis of post-transplant lymphoproliferative disorder in solid organ transplant recipients - BCSH and BTS Guidelines. *Br J Haematol* 2010;149(5):675–92.

Chapter 12

Fertility, contraception, and pregnancy

Frank P Edenborough

Key points

Males

- Most likely to be infertile—counsel early and do a sperm test at around 18 years
- Fatherhood is possible using sperm retrieval and *in vitro* fertilization (MESA and ICSI)

Females

- Menarche is likely to be delayed but regular menses are the norm unless in poor health
- All women of reproductive age should be considered fertile and offered contraception
- True fertility is unknown, but up to two-thirds of women wishing to become pregnant do so naturally
- The outcome for the mother is highly dependent on her pre-conceptual health, notably weight and lung function
- For those unable to conceive, bypassing the cervical mucus plug (intrauterine insemination) or more formal *in vitro* fertilization techniques are available

Pregnancy

- The outcome of pregnancy for the child is generally excellent
- Maintaining the mother's health with full usual CF treatment far outweighs the risk to the baby from potential fetal drug toxicity
- The risk of the child having CF depends on the partner's carrier status
- The fetus can be tested by chorionic villus sampling or amniocentesis, or in IVF a healthy embryo can be selected by pre-implantation genetic diagnosis
- Pregnancy after lung transplant is possible but there is increased risk of transplant rejection, and obstetric complications including eclampsia and fetal prematurity

12.1 **Introduction**

Over half the UK CF population (57% of 10 078, 2012) are over 16 and likely to be taking an active interest in sexual and reproductive health. Evidence suggests high proportions are in long-term relationships and many already have children. However, many young adults are poorly educated regarding their reproductive potential and contraception is often poorly understood. Pregnancy is possible in the healthy woman but accidental pregnancy in a sick woman may be disastrous. Subfertility remains an issue for many with CF, especially men wishing to father their own children, but *in vitro* fertilization (IVF) techniques can help both sexes become biological parents.

12.2 **Growth and puberty**

Historically, people with CF were on average shorter and lighter than non-CF individuals. This was assumed to be due to poor nutrition, but it remains true today despite optimum nutrition. CFTR has been found in the hypothalamus and elsewhere in the brain, suggesting it may also have a role in central hormonal control. However, the hypothalamic–pituitary–gonadal axis produces normal hormone levels, and although puberty in men and women is delayed by up to 2 years, secondary sexual characteristics are normal. Ill health results in reduced levels of insulin and insulin-like growth factors (IGF1, IGF-BP3), which have some gonadotrophin-like properties. Growth and puberty are significantly impaired in those with CF related diabetes (CFRD).

12.2.1 **The effect of CFTR on reproductive tissues**

Males

CFTR is found in the epididymis, vas deferens, seminal vesicles, and ejaculatory ducts from as early as 18 weeks *in utero*. In CF, these structures are usually obstructed, atretic, or absent at birth.

- 98% of men will have obstructive azoospermia and be infertile
- Congenital bilateral absence of the vas deferens (CBAVD) is seen even in mild forms of CF suggesting these structures are particularly sensitive to CFTR dysfunction
- Many infertile men with CBAVD (responsible for 1–2% of male infertility) may have at least one CF mutation or indeed subclinical CF themselves
- The most frequent genotype in this context (40%) is ΔF508/R117H 9T/5T (functionally significant 5T variant of the polythymidine tract at intron 8)

Females

The cervix, endometrium, and fallopian tubes all express CFTR but are anatomically normal.

- Cervical goblet cell hyperplasia may lead to viscid mucus unresponsive to hormonal change at ovulation ('ferning'), and causing obstruction of the cervical os by a mucus plug, resulting in subfertility
- The ovaries and breast tissues are unaffected by CFTR

The female cycle

Menarche is on average delayed by up to 2 years (mean age ~14). Primary amenorrhoea (no periods at age 16) is rare, but irregular cycles, anovulatory cycles with follicular cysts and secondary amenorrhoea are commonly associated with episodes of ill health and may be temporary.

12.3 Sexual development and contraception

12.3.1 Sexual function and fertility

Surveys of patients and their parents that indicated that both parties are often poorly informed about CF reproductive issues and would like to be informed by their CF teams, girls by age 12–13 and boys by age 14. Healthcare providers are often uncomfortable discussing issues of sexual health, but unplanned pregnancy can be a disaster and may be considered a failure of care if such discussions have not taken place.

Males

Men with CF have normal sex hormone levels, normal virilization, and normal libido, but some are upset reading about infertility due to confusion with impotence. Whilst 98% are likely to be infertile, potency is not affected (although some notice the ejaculate is thin, watery, acidic, and of small volume), and it is generally felt that information on infertility with clarification that sexual function is normal should be given during transition to adult services.

- Azoospermia should be checked for after age 18 (because there are no normative values for younger men) during periods of good health and after sexual abstinence for 3–4 days

Females

Coitarche in women with CF is at the same age as in non-CF. Sexual function is normal although vaginal dryness and thrush (associated with antibiotics, steroids, and diabetes) is more common and may be associated with dyspareunia.

The potential fertility of women with CF is unknown as many choose not to have children, but studies report success rates of around two-thirds of women wishing to conceive doing so without recourse to assisted reproductive techniques (ART).

12.3.2 Contraception

Contraceptive efficacy assuming correct use are given in brackets.

Males

Men should not assume that they are infertile until they have had a sperm test.

- All men with CF should use a condom (98% efficacy) for all casual sexual encounters to prevent sexually transmitted diseases

Females

Even with advanced lung disease, CF women can conceive and all should receive contraceptive advice.

- The range of contraceptive choices for women with CF is as for non-CF women
- Only condoms (98% efficacy), and the femidom (95%), protect against sexually transmitted diseases

1. *Barrier contraceptives*

    - The cap or diaphragm (92–96%) should be used in conjunction with spermicidal cream

2. *Oral contraceptives (98% efficacy)*

    - Combined oestrogen-/progestogen-containing pills (cyclical, permitting menses) should contain at least 30 micrograms oestrogen

- Progesterone-only pills prevent menstruation but may be complicated by break-through bleeding and may potentiate osteopenia

Potential complications

There is a theoretical risk of reduced absorption during new antibiotic courses. Barrier precautions are recommended during and for 7 days after antibiotic treatment. Increased sputum viscosity, reduced lung function, impaired liver function and glycaemic control, and thrombogenesis in the context of implantable venous access devices, are all theoretical risks and should be monitored for at least the first 6 months. Further, some drugs interact with oestrogen-containing pills.

3. *Medium-acting combined oestrogen/progestogen devices*
   - The Evra® transdermal patch changed weekly for 3 weeks with a patch-free week may be considered, but caution is suggested on sticking to CF skin
   - The Nuvaring® vaginal ring is inserted for 3 weeks, removed for a week, and a new ring inserted next cycle

4. *Long-acting reversible methods*
   - Injectable contraceptives (>99% efficacy)

     Long-acting progestogens can be given IM (Depo-Provera®) or as implanted rods (Nexplanon®/Implanon®) in those for whom the pill is unsuitable. Both may be associated with break-through bleeding and osteopenia. Nexplanon®/Implanon® may be more suitable for long-term use with less osteopenia and quicker return of ovulation on removal
   - Intrauterine devices (IUDs) (98–99% effective rate)

     May contain copper or elute progesterone (e.g. the levonorgestrel intrauterine system (IUS) Mirena® coil changed 5-yearly). Modern systems are suitable for nulliparous women but should be discussed with, and inserted by, a specialist

5. *Tubal ligation*
   - This may be considered in someone decidedly against having a child, someone with a child who wishes to have no more, or in someone too ill to consider a future pregnancy who is struggling with other contraceptive means. This may include vasectomy for the partner

---

Key point

Pregnancy has been in reported in severely underweight CF women on transplant lists. Outcomes are usually poor for the mother, whether the pregnancy is completed or termination is performed. All women with CF should be considered fertile and adequate contraception offered.

12.4 **Reproductive genetics and counselling**

- CF is an autosomal recessive state and all gametes will have an abnormal CF gene; i.e. all offspring will be (at least) carriers
- The risk of someone with CF having a CF child is entirely dependent on the partner. If the partner is a carrier then the risk is 1:2. If untested (based on European carrier frequency of 1:25), the risk is 1:50, and if tested and not a carrier, the risk is less than 1:700

12.4.1 Genetic counselling

Ideally, discussions with the couple should start well before conception. The nature of CF, the unaffected carrier status, and whether wider family members should be informed if a gene is identified in the partner should all be discussed. The specific risks of vertical transmission, implications of potential subfertility, the potential effect of CF on the pregnancy and child, and the effect of pregnancy on the woman with CF, should all be explored.

12.4.2 Psychological counselling

People with CF generally wish to live a normal life, and many will want to have a family. Some girls, whether in a relationship or not, express a desire to leave something of themselves behind. Sub/infertility may be devastating news to a person with CF wishing to have a child. Perhaps worse is when a woman is advised she should not become pregnant because she is too unwell to either conceive or carry a pregnancy, or when an accidentally pregnant woman with advanced CF is told that a therapeutic termination may be the only way to save her. Couples should be advised:

- of the potential effect of CF on the pregnancy and the unborn child AND of the potential long-term effect of the pregnancy on the mother's health
- to consider finances, family support for childcare to enable the mother to rest and undergo treatment, and the question of who can help at the time of illness or hospitalization
- that there is a reasonable chance the partner with CF may become too sick to participate in childcare and may not survive long enough to see their child reach adulthood

Many multidisciplinary CF teams have psychologists on the team who are best placed to explore these issues.

12.5 Assisted conception

12.5.1 Assisted conception techniques

Males

Although the ejaculate is azoospermic and spermatogenesis and sperm maturation may be impaired, sufficient sperm can usually be retrieved from the testes and caput medusa and used with artificial reproductive techniques. PESA (percutaneous epididymal sperm aspiration), TESA and TESE, (testicular sperm aspiration/extraction by biopsy) can yield sufficient sperm of good quality even in ill health to facilitate pregnancy by intracytoplasmic sperm injection (ICSI).

To optimize the chance of a pregnancy, the (healthy) partner of a man with CF will have to undergo investigation and treatment similar to those of a CF woman trying to conceive (see Box 12.1).

Females

In healthy women with CF who cannot conceive, the most likely cause is a cervical mucus plug which can be by-passed by intrauterine sperm injection (IUI). However, many women less well with CF will have difficulty conceiving and they will require full investigation and undergo *in vitro* fertilization techniques (IVF) (see Box 12.1).

> ### Box 12.1 *In vitro* fertilization
>
> Assuming a woman is otherwise reasonably well with her CF, IVF is usually considered if baseline tests are normal (including hormone profile, pelvic and transvaginal ultrasound, and possibly hysterosalpingogram for tubal patency). Superovulation is induced by follicle-stimulating hormone (FSH), ova are 'ripened' with human chorionic gonadotrophin (HCG) and developing follicles are monitored by ultrasound and oestradiol levels. These are harvested 34–38 hrs later by transvaginal follicular aspiration under sedation. Fertilization is achieved by incubation with washed sperm for 48–72 hrs or by ICSI. Embryo transfer by intrauterine injection occurs at the 6–8 cell stage on day 2 or 3 post fertilization. Pregnancy rates of up to 50% per cycle can be expected, with live birth rates of 40% under the age of 35, declining with increased maternal age.

- Pregnancy is unlikely in the very underweight (BMI <18 kg/m^2) or in those with secondary amenorrhoea due to significant pulmonary or hepatic disease. These women are unlikely to be considered for IVF

12.5.2 **Genetic testing of the fetus**

When a woman with CF presents already pregnant and the father's genotype cannot be tested or he is a carrier of an identifiable gene, chorionic villus sampling (8–12 weeks) or amniocentesis (12–18 weeks) can be performed to test to see whether the fetus has CF. If the partner is found to be a carrier prior to conception, pre-implantation genetic diagnosis (PGD) is possible by taking a cell from the developing embryo (day 3–5) and testing for CF. Couples may choose to have only a healthy (carrier) embryo implanted, avoiding the risk of miscarriage with CVS (1–2%) or amniocentesis (1%).

> ### Key point
>
> Current CF genotype-testing techniques are limited and do not reduce the risk of a CF child to zero because some genes cannot be routinely identified prior to conception or with CVS/amniocentesis. CF may yet be diagnosed in the infant on clinical grounds and by sweat testing.

12.6 **Pregnancy in women with CF**

12.6.1 **Background**

The first pregnancy in a woman with CF was reported in 1960. Subsequent cases and annual reports from the North American CF Database confirmed pregnancy was increasingly common (currently 3–4% of women over the age of 17). Early reviews suggested pregnancy was only likely to succeed in healthy women with CF (late diagnosis, pancreatic-sufficient, good weight and lung function, no diabetes). Increasingly, pregnancy is seen in pancreatic-insufficient women, and there are numerous reports of women surviving pregnancy despite impaired lung function.

- In general, healthy women can expect a normal pregnancy, aiming for normal vaginal delivery at term with the opportunity to breastfeed the infant thereafter

- In those less well, poor weight, or weight gain in pregnancy, and poor lung function all predict the likelihood of increased respiratory exacerbations, increased hospital visits, intensification of treatment, and a propensity to premature delivery via assisted delivery techniques (due to maternal concerns) whether planned or as an emergency

> **Key point**
>
> While some women report their best-ever health in pregnancy, even healthy women may experience a faster than expected decline in their CF health, and may not fully recover after delivery.

12.6.2 Preparing for pregnancy

Counselling

Risks of pregnancy, covering topics including whether pregnancy is right for the woman? Who will care for child or for her if she is ill? Survival with child, and fitting treatment around childcare.

Genetic counselling

Make sure that the partner is offered testing.

Optimize medication

Advise continuation of all routine CF medication. Avoid starting new medication peri-conception. Recommend full treatment of any chest infection before contraception stops. (N.B. no evidence of teratogenicity of any CF therapies to-date)

- Start folic acid 400 mcg and continue to 14 weeks

- Check vitamin A levels and continue usual supplemental dose (<10 000 IU/day) unless high/low levels (both associated with teratogenicity)

- Check iron and consider supplementation if low

Optimize nutrition

Aim for pre-conception body weight >90% ideal.

- Plan for 300+ kcal extra a day (up to 150% recommended daily requirements)

- Consider energy-dense foods, oral supplements, or early instigation of nasogastric or gastrostomy (difficult to do in late pregnancy), tube feeding

- Aim for weight gain of at least 10 kg during pregnancy (more if underweight)

Physiotherapy

Optimize airway clearance and review adherence, technique, sequence, and necessity of inhaled medication and exercise regimens.

- Breathlessness in the first trimester is hormonally driven and women should be advised this is likely, but beware infection

- In late pregnancy, the expanding uterus compresses basal areas of the lungs increasing the risk of sputum trapping and infection

- Unlike non-CF pregnancies, there is frequently a decline in FEV_1 and FVC as pregnancy progresses

- General cardiovascular fitness, core stability, and strength is important
- Pelvic floor exercises should be encouraged. Cough-urinary incontinence is common in girls with CF and is likely to get worse during and after pregnancy (see Chapter 9)

12.6.3 *Monitoring during pregnancy*

Lung function, weight, and glucose homeostasis should be monitored carefully throughout pregnancy.

- Women should probably be seen bimonthly until ~32 weeks, then monthly until 38 weeks, and weekly thereafter (remember to try and coincide/ liaise with obstetric visits)
- Gestational diabetes is relatively common in CF pregnancy (up to 40%), and will generally require insulin. Approximately 50% resolve post partum but some will progress to CF related diabetes (CFRD)
- Blood sugar should be measured on each visit, particularly during exacerbations
- Oral glucose tolerance tests, routinely done in pregnancy at 20 weeks, should be performed at onset of pregnancy, at 20 weeks, 28 weeks, or if there is any doubt

12.6.4 **Management of CF during pregnancy**

Respiratory exacerbation and declining lung function with hypoxia pose the greatest threat to mother and hence to baby. Any decline should be treated aggressively with review of airway clearance, bronchodilators, oral antibiotics, and a low threshold for intravenous antibiotics, and with supplemental oxygen if SaO_2 falls below 94%.

- Conventional dual antibiotic therapy with a β-lactam and aminoglycoside (with close monitoring of levels) is safe. There are no reports of fetal ototoxicty in mothers treated with these regimens and the risk to the baby from hypoxia or sepsis far outweighs the potential risk from drug therapy
- Poor weight gain should be investigated by reviewing actual calorie/ nutrient intake, enzyme usage, and instigation of oral, tube, or even parenteral feeding should be considered early, especially if gastrostomy feeding likely
- Be vigilant for pregnancy-related hyperemesis gravidarum, reflux, and dyspepsia, and constipation (or worsening CF-related distal obstruction symptoms)
- The onset of gestational diabetes should be treated with maintained high-calorie intake covered by insulin

12.6.5 **Obstetric considerations in CF pregnancy**

As soon as pregnancy is confirmed, close liaison must begin with the obstetric and CF teams. This includes between the CF specialist nurse and midwives, and between the CF physician and obstetrician, and an anaesthetist familiar with high-risk obstetric cases. Visits should coincide to reduce inconvenience to the mother and avoid duplication of tests.

- The incidence of obstetric complications is not increased in CF. Occasional bleeding, hypertension, and similar rates of tubal pregnancy and miscarriage to the non-CF population have been reported
- Most problems encountered will have an origin in the mother's CF health; namely, poor maternal weight gain and intrauterine growth retardation (not a feature of CF per se)

- Early discussion with the mother must consider preferred analgesia and mode of delivery, but must also cover the possibility of planned or emergency early intervention and delivery if either mother or baby is in crisis
- Approximately 25% of deliveries may be premature (<37weeks), usually necessitated by deteriorating maternal lung function

Analgesia

Epidural anaesthesia early in stage 1 of delivery gives good analgesia, saves energy for stage 2 (delivery), and facilitates natural childbirth, but can be converted to spinal anaesthesia for instrumentation or caesarean section if required. It can also be left in situ to allow early mobilization and chest physiotherapy after delivery.

Mode and timing of delivery

Whilst normal vaginal delivery at term is the outcome of choice, some women may choose Caesarean section and others may be too unwell to manage natural childbirth without assistance. The obstetrician and physician may plan for early induction at or before 40 weeks where the mother is struggling or if the baby is big (macrosomia with diabetes) or the mother is small (due to CF). In advanced CF or in the context of severe decline in pregnancy, steroids may be given to prepare the fetal lungs with planned delivery any time after 32 weeks, or in the eventuality of an emergency delivery.

12.6.6 **Breastfeeding**

'Breast is best' (for the baby), even in CF, since breast-milk composition is essentially normal. Breastfeeding, however, requires up to an additional 500 kcal day and may be hard for a CF mother to sustain. Formula-feed supplementation may be necessary but breastfeeding should be encouraged for at least 3 weeks.

12.6.7 **CF-related drugs and pregnancy**

Most drugs used routinely in CF are safe in pregnancy. Enzymes, PPIs, vitamins (check vitamin A levels and use <10 000 IU day), all inhaled drugs including antibiotics should be continued. Ursodeoxycholic acid (see Chapter 14) should be avoided in the first trimester, so ideally stopped before conception when the pregnancy is planned. Penicillins and macrolides are safe, tetracyclines, chloramphenicol, and co-trimoxazole should be avoided, and ciprofloxacin used with caution. Intravenous (IV) piperacillin/ tazobactam, ceftazidime, meropenem, and aztreonam are safe. Once-daily tobramycin with careful measurement of levels can be used but consider risk–benefit as there is a small risk of fetal nephro- or ototoxicity. IV colistimethate sodium should probably be avoided.

Drugs acting on CFTR function

The recently introduced ivacaftor is a specific activator of the class III mutation G551D. Taken orally, its effects are seen widely with improved lung function, weight, and significant correction of sweat chloride (see Chapter 4). Patients report greater well-being, and anecdotally, some women who have long tried for a pregnancy have become pregnant shortly after starting it, presumably by correction of the cervical mucus gland function. It is unlicensed and untested in pregnancy and its excretion in breast milk is unknown. Consequently it is not advised in pregnancy. Contraception is recommended and the drug stopped if pregnancy contemplated. However, it is FDA Category B rated. There are no adequate, well controlled studies in human pregnancy and no risk has been shown to the fetus in animal studies. <http://www.accessdata.fda.gov/drugsatfda_docs/label/2012/203188lbl.pdf>. Whilst ivacaftor cannot be recommended, it appears to be so effective in CF that women may choose to continue to take it. Pragmatic clinical advice might be to stop it pre-conception (or as soon as pregnancy is suspected) and restart after pregnancy if the mother is well; stop it as above but restart in the third trimester if the mother is struggling; or continue throughout if the mother has more advanced CF and had made a clinical improvement when the drug was commenced. There are anecdotal reports of successful pregnancies in each of the above scenarios and no evidence of teratogenicity to date.

12.6.8 **Pregnancy after transplantation**

Many women who undergo successful lung transplantation see it as a second chance and consider the opportunity to have a child. Many successful pregnancies have been reported in solid-organ transplants including kidney, liver, and heart. However, there is less experience of pregnancy after heart and lung, or double-lung transplant.

* Successful pregnancies have been reported but there is a high incidence of eclampsia, prematurity, and graft rejection
* Pregnancy seems to exacerbate rejection (despite up-titration of therapy to account for increased volume of distribution)
* General advice remains cautious

> Key point
>
> Pregnancy is not recommended within 2 years of transplantation or if there have been significant episodes of rejection or declining lung function since transplant.

12.6.9 **Fetal outcome in CF pregnancy**

Early studies suggested increased perinatal mortality but this is no longer the case due to advances in obstetric and paediatric care and special-care baby units. Fetal prematurity is declining and birth weight increasing despite a tendency for mothers to be older and have less good lung function than historically. This is often at a cost of increased treatment and hospital stay during pregnancy.

* Fetal anomalies have been reported in CF pregnancies but none have been attributed to either CF, its treatment, or transplant-related treatment
* No long-term studies have been performed on babies to CF parents, and the potential for physical or psychological sequelae as a consequence of having a sick parent or of losing a parent during childhood remain unknown

12.6.10 **Maternal outcomes in CF pregnancy**

Since early reports appeared in the literature it has been clear that some women with CF do badly during pregnancy, experiencing catastrophic change in lung function and weight that is not recovered in the post-partum years. Maternal survival with child is often poor. What is not clear is whether these women were likely to do badly even if they were not pregnant. The markers of poor outcome for pregnancy in CF are the same as for poor outcome for CF generally. Case-control comparisons of pregnant versus age and severity matched non-pregnant controls are dominated by the only large and adequately statistically powered study from the North American database.

* Women who became pregnant were healthier than those who did not

- Women who became pregnant had better survival overall
- When the data was corrected for disease severity, even women with FEV_1 <40% appeared to do better than equivalent non-pregnant controls
- The group most at risk was those women who conceived when very young (<18)
- Initial concerns regarding loss of lung function during pregnancy and not recovered post partum and of rapid weight loss post partum have been ameliorated to some extent by modern management

Key point

It is worth considering that 20% of mothers will die before their child's 10th birthday, and if FEV_1<40%, 40% will die before child's 10th birthday.

12.6.11 **Contra-indications to pregnancy**

The only absolute contra-indications remain pulmonary hypertension and cor pulmonale. Relative contra-indications are FEV_1<60%, BMI<18, CF-related diabetes, and infection with *B. cenocepacia*.

12.6.12 **Termination of pregnancy in CF**

Termination of pregnancy may be requested for accidental pregnancy for psychosocial reasons or may be necessitated by poor maternal health or for obstetric reasons, e.g. anomalies.

- Medical termination using oral mifepristone followed by prostaglandin vaginally or by mouth avoids the need for anaesthesia and instrumentation
- Surgical termination may be necessary as determined by the obstetrician

Summary

Males

- Most likely to be infertile—counsel early and do a sperm test at ~age 18
- Advise condom use in case one of the 2% without azoospermia and to protect against sexually transmitted disease
- Fatherhood is possible using sperm retrieval and *in vitro* fertilization (MESA and ICSI)
- Success rates are up to 50% per cycle
- The risk of a child with CF depends on the partner's carrier status

Females

- Menarche is likely to be delayed but regular menses are the norm unless in poor health
- All women of reproductive age should be considered fertile and offered contraception
- Only condoms and femidoms protect against sexually transmitted diseases
- True fertility is unknown but up to two-thirds of women wishing to become pregnant do so naturally

- The outcome of pregnancy for the child is excellent
- The outcome for the mother is highly dependent on her pre-conceptual health, notably weight and lung function
- For those unable to conceive, by passing the cervical mucus plug (intrauterine insemination), or more formal *in vitro* fertilization techniques are available
- The risk of a child with CF depends on the partner's carrier status
- The fetus can be tested by chorionic villus sampling or amniocentesis or in IVF a healthy embryo can be selected by pre-implantation genetic diagnosis if the partner is a carrier
- Maintaining the mother's health with full usual CF treatment far outweighs the risk to the baby from potential fetal drug toxicity
- Pregnancy after transplantation should probably be delayed for 2 years and counselled against if there have been significant episodes of rejection prior to conception

References

Edenborough FP. Guidelines for the management of pregnancy in women with cystic fibrosis. *J Cyst Fibrosis* 2008;7,S2:1–32.

Goss CH. The effect of pregnancy on survival in women with *Cystic Fibrosis Chest* 2003;124:1460–8.

Gyi KM. Pregnancy in cystic fibrosis lung transplant recipients: case series and review. *J Cyst Fibrosis* 2006;5:171–6.

Smith H.C. (2010). Fertility in men with cystic fibrosis. Assessment, investigations and management. *Paediatric Respiratory Reviews* 11, 80–83.

Thorpe-Beeston JG. Contraception and pregnancy in cystic fibrosis. *J Royal Soc Med* 2009;102:S3–S10.

Tsang A. Contraception, communication and counseling for sexuality and reproductive health in adolescents and young adults with CF. *Paediatric Respiratory Reviews* 2010;11:84–9.

Chapter 13

Future treatments

Rebecca Thursfield, Chris Orchard, Rosanna Featherstone,
and Jane C Davies

Key points

- Increased understanding of CF pathophysiology has led to further developments in new treatments
- The CFTR potentiator, ivacaftor, is now licensed for patients with class III (gating) mutations. In combinations with the corrector, Lumacaftor, it also led to clinical improvement in patients homozygous for Phe508del. Additional CFTR correctors are also now being trialled
- The UK CF Gene Therapy Consortium is concluding a large phase 2b repeated dose randomized placebo-controlled trial of cationic liposome-mediated CFTR gene therapy, to determine clinical efficacy
- Non-specific methods of rehydrating the airway surface via ion transport-targeted therapies have been successful, and both hypertonic saline and mannitol are now in use in the clinical setting
- Developments in infection include novel antibiotic design, delivery by alternative routes, targeting bacterial biofilms, and alternatives to conventional antimicrobials, such as bacteriophage and immunity-based strategies

For decades, the treatment of CF has been symptomatic, tackling the downstream consequences of the disease, such as airway infection, rather than its root cause. The last couple of years have brought with them the promise that this is about to change, with the first licensed CFTR modulator for a small proportion of the CF population. The demonstration with trials of this drug that CFTR is a useful therapeutic target has re-energized the field of drug development for CF. Here we review the pipeline and present an update on future directions. Where trials are ongoing, the NCT number represents that study's National Clinical Trial number on the *clinicaltrials.gov* trial registration website.

13.1 CFTR gene therapy

Since the discovery of the *CFTR* gene, numerous attempts have been made to reverse the basic defect by gene transfer. Laboratory tests demonstrated successful restoration of ion transport with either modified viral vectors or synthetic gene transfer techniques, but achieving similar success in the clinic has been challenging. The majority of clinical trials have been single-dose, proof-of-concept design, often administering the gene therapy to the nasal epithelium for ease of access for delivery and assays. Whilst most trials have reported both transgene expression based on mRNA levels and electrophysiological correction of nasal potential difference (NPD), the results have largely been variable and of short duration. Attempts to dose repeatedly have confirmed that currently the majority of viral vectors lead to immune responses which limit efficacy upon subsequent administration. Furthermore, clinical efficacy remains to be determined. The UK CF Gene Therapy Consortium <http://www.cfgenetherapy.org.uk/> is currently concluding a large, phase 2b, repeated dose, randomized placebo-controlled trial of cationic liposome-mediated *CFTR* gene therapy. Nebulized doses have been administered at monthly intervals over 1 year, with a primary outcome of change in FEV$_1$. Secondary outcomes include lung clearance index (LCI), CT scans, validated quality-of-life questionnaires, inflammatory markers, and electrophysiological assessments. In parallel to this clinical programme, the Consortium is developing a second-wave product, a pseudotyped lentivirus, which unlike most viral vectors appears to be repeatedly administrable. The advantages of this approach are high levels of transfection and the potential for very long duration of expression, which may allow extremely infrequent dosing. This approach will require detailed preclinical toxicity testing and optimization before clinical trials commence.

13.2 **Mutation-specific CFTR modulators**

As described in Chapter 1, over 1900 different mutations have been identified in the *CFTR* gene. These fall into one of 6 classes depending on their functional impact on CFTR protein (see Chapter 1, Figure 1.8). Three treatment approaches are being explored based on our knowledge of these classes:

1 Read-through of premature truncation codons (class 1 mutations)

2 'Corrector' agents which allow misfolded CFTR protein to be trafficked to the cell surface (class 2 mutations)

3 'Potentiators' which increase the open probability of CFTR protein (initially licenced for class 3 mutations, but effective against many other CFTR forms, including wild type)

13.2.1 **Class 1 mutations**

Often termed 'nonsense' or 'stop' mutations, these contain a premature termination codon (PTC) which results in a short and unstable mRNA and non-functional CFTR protein. Examples of class I mutations include Trp1282X (previously W1282X) and Gly542X. They are highly prevalent amongst the Jewish CF population, and account for 60% of CF in Israel. Worldwide, class I mutations account for 5–10% of the CF population.

Following the discovery that certain drugs, such as gentamicin, could allow the ribosome to 'skip' the stop mutation and lead to full-length protein, ataluren (PTC124), a compound with similar properties but a more favourable toxicity profile has been developed and trialed both in CF and in stop-mutation-mediated Duchenne muscular dystrophy. This orally bioavailable molecule, administered 3 times daily as a dose-adjusted powder, showed promise in early phase trials. However, in a recent large, multinational, phase 3, randomized double blind, placebo-controlled trial of adults and children (Kerem et al., 2014) neither primary (change in FEV$_1$) nor multiple secondary outcomes were met for the group as a whole. Fascinatingly, a pre-specified post-hoc subgroup analysis did demonstrate a significant effect of the co-administration of nebulized tobramycin, with those patients not exposed to this drug showing a significant treatment effect. A further trial to examine this more closely is being conducted.

13.2.2 **Correctors**

The observation that culture at low temperature allowed misfolded ΔF508 CFTR to traffic to the cell surface where it functioned (albeit not to wild-type levels) led to a concerted effort to identify drugs capable of 'correcting' this mutation. To-date, 2 of these, both produced by Vertex Pharmaceuticals, have reached the clinical trial stage. Lumacaftor (VX-809) significantly improved chloride transport in ΔF508 CFTR cells *in vitro* to 14% of non-CF levels.

However, a phase 2 study of VX-809 monotherapy in 89 homozygous adults demonstrated only a very small (7 mmol/L) reduction in sweat chloride, and no change in nasal potential difference, sweat chloride, or clinical status. The interesting prospect of combining such drugs with potentiators does, however, seem to be coming of age. *In vitro*, the addition of ivacaftor to lumacaftor led to a significant increase in chloride secretion, and in early groups of an ongoing phase 2 study of this combination (NCT01225211), significant improvements in FEV_1 have been reported. This has led to a large phase 3 programme (clinicaltrials.gov trial numbers: NCT01807923 and NCT01807949), which recruited over 1000 ΔF508 homozygous patients aged 12 and above worldwide. Although not published at the time of writing, conference presentations (NACFC 2014) have reported a significant improvement in FEV_1 and frequency of pulmonary exacerbations.

A second corrector compound (VX-661; NCT01531673) is currently in phase 2 studies in combination with ivacaftor. Other small molecule correctors are also being explored by several other companies. However, recent recognition that at least two different misfolding steps may need to be independently corrected illustrates the huge task ahead.

13.2.3 Potentiators

Class 3 mutations, of which the commonest is Gly551Asp (also known as G551D), lead to normally positioned protein which fails to open in response to ATP binding and leads to markedly reduced chloride conductance. High throughput screening identified several small molecules which facilitated opening and have been termed potentiators. The lead molecule, VX-770, was shown *in-vitro* to increase chloride secretion, airway surface liquid height, and ciliary function. This agent was fast-tracked into clinical development and is now the first in class CFTR modulator, and known as ivacaftor. Phase 3 trial data showed significant improvements in lung function, exacerbation rate, weight gain, and quality of life in addition to the biomarker sweat chloride, and the drug is now approved in the US, EU, and Australasia for patients aged 6 years and over with at least one copy of G551D (see Chapter 4). In addition, a recent phase 3 trial has confirmed similar efficacy in non-G551D class 3 mutations, a safety trial is underway in younger children (NCT01705145), and the drug has been studied in patients with the class 4 conductance defect, R117H (NCT01614457).

13.3 Ion transport-targeted therapies

Non-specific methods of rehydrating the airway surface have been successful and both hypertonic saline and mannitol are now in the clinic (see Chapter 4). Various attempts have been made in the past to target directly non-CFTR ion channels (eg. the P2Y2 agonist denufosol) but to-date this has met with limited success and/or inconsistent results. No trials of agents in this category are currently listed in the drug development pipeline of the US Cystic Fibrosis Foundation <http://www.cff.org/research/drugdevelopmentpipeline/>.

13.4 Anti-inflammatory agents

The CF inflammatory response appears exaggerated, prolonged, and incompletely effective. Although controversy remains over whether this is due to a primary defect or whether it occurs only after an infective trigger, data from the CF pig model would support the latter. The oral non-steroidal anti-inflammatory agent, ibuprofen, is widely used in the US but seldom in Europe, largely due to concerns over level monitoring and side effects. Although there is little direct proof from clinical trials, the anti-inflammatory properties of macrolide antibiotics may be responsible for at least some of the clinical benefits of azithromycin.

The CFF drug-development pipeline currently lists 2 agents in phase 2 trials in this category: nebulized $\alpha_1$antitrypsin and the phosphodiesterase inhibitor, sildenafil. The last trial of an anti-inflammatory agent in CF (BIIL284; Konstan et al., 2014#2) highlighted the potential downsides of abrogating a bacterial-targeted host defence response as it had to be terminated early due to an increased number of infective exacerbations in the actively treated arm.

13.5 **Antimicrobial strategies**

Although the aggressive use of conventional antibiotics has undoubtedly been responsible for much of the improved health of today's patients, there are significant problems including the emergence of newer organisms, antimicrobial multi-drug resistance, allergies, and toxicities including renal and auditory nerve damage. Developments in this field include: a) attempts to design novel antibiotic agents, b) reformulation of current drugs for improved delivery, e.g. nebulized formulations of intravenous preparations and dry powder in place of nebulized solutions, c) targeting bacterial biofilms, and d) alternatives to conventional antimicrobials such as bacteriophage and immunity-based strategies. These can most easily be discussed with reference to the major CF pathogen, *Pseudomonas aeruginosa*. This organism is the most prevalent chronic infection in the CF airway. It possesses an armamentarium of defences against host and administered antimicrobials, one of the major strategies being the development of biofilms (see Chapter 3).

Conventional antibiotics

Currently, conventional anti-pseudomonal antibiotics are administered orally, topically, or systemically, the latter usually being reserved for periods of infective exacerbation. In the last few years, both colomycin and tobramycin have been reformulated into dry powders with no apparent loss of efficacy, and nebulized aztreonam has become available. In terms of newer developments, Arikace™ is a sustained-release, liposomal formulation of amikacin for inhalation, the advantages of which include greater penetration into the biofilm, and site-specific release of drug from the liposomes by bacterial rhamnolipids. Phase 2 placebo-controlled trials demonstrated significant improvements in FEV_1, *Pa* density, exacerbation rate, and time to rescue antibiotics. A phase 3 trial has recently begun in which Arikace™ will be compared with TOBI on a month on/month off basis (NCT01315678), and there is also interest in a similar approach for *Mycobacterium abscessus* and *Staphylococcus aureus*. A novel formulation of levofloxacin (MP-376, Aeroquin®/Quinsair®) has been developed. A recent, multicentre, randomized, dose-ranging study of MP-376 in 151 patients found the optimum dose was 240 mg BD, and this led to an 8.7% increase in FEV_1 compared with placebo. Significant reductions in the need for other anti-pseudomonal antibiotics were observed in all treatment groups, and it was well tolerated. Two phase 3 trials of Aeroquin®/Quinsair® are currently ongoing (NCT01180634, NCT01270347).

Ciprofloxacin is currently being studied in several formulations for inhalation. A phase 2 trial of ciprofloxacin alone has been completed and the results are awaited (NCT00645788). A further proof-of-concept trial of dry powder ciprofloxacin in combination with dornase alfa has been carried out.

Fosfomycin in combination with tobramycin (FTI), has been tested in a placebo-controlled multicentre study and showed promise in terms of lung function, *Pa* density, MRSA, and *S.aureus*. Further trials will be needed to confirm safety and efficacy.

13.5.1 **Antibody-based approaches**

Active immunization against *Pa* has met with limited success, but several approaches based on passive immunization are still being explored. Immunoglobulin (Ig)Y is present in high levels in the yolks of hens' eggs; specific antibacterial IgYs can be generated by immunization of the hens. A small, open-label study of prophylactic treatment with anti-pseudomonal IgY was performed in Sweden. Seventeen patients were given daily IgY solution, which was gargled and then swallowed. They were matched with a control group receiving standard treatment in Danish centres. The treatment group had lower rates of positive *Pa* cultures, and lower rates of chronic colonization. A multicentre, phase 3 randomized controlled trial has recently begun in Europe (NCT01455675). Work is also being carried out on a humanized monoclonal Fab fragment that targets a *Pa* virulence factor (Type III secretion system) called KB001. Currently a phase 2 randomized controlled trial is being carried out and the results are awaited (NCT00638365).

13.5.2 **Biofilm-targeted approaches**

Quorum sensing (QS) is an intercellular communication system in which *Pa* actively senses the concentration of neighbouring bacteria, and when a threshold is reached, the genes leading to biofilm formation will be switched on. Inhibition of QS could therefore be a viable approach to reduce biofilm formation and allow more effective use of antibiotics. One of the major modes of action of the macrolide antibiotic, azithromycin, appears to be quorum sensing inhibition. A pilot study using garlic as a QS inhibitor has recently been carried out, without any significant change in outcome, but further trials are planned. In addition to previously known inhibitors, many laboratories are performing high-throughput screens in an attempt to find analogues for clinical use. The observation that nitrites and related molecules can both kill mucoid *Pseudomonas* (*Pa*) and lead to disruption of biofilms may lead to future clinically applicable developments.

13.5.3 **Bacteriophage**

Bacteriophages are viruses which can bind to and infect bacteria but not eukaryotic cells. They have been used for many decades in certain parts of the world, but have largely not been subjected to well-designed trials. Lytic phages enter their bacterial host, amplify and lyse the bacteria, releasing progeny phages which can quickly outnumber their host bacteria. In theory, this has several advantages: they could be complementary to existing antimicrobial therapy, currently available data suggest low toxicity, and previously resistant bacterial strains may be susceptible to treatment with phage. Some of the obstacles to phage-based treatment have been overcome and, as interest increases, not only for CF but a multitude of bacterial diseases, trials have been conducted in tightly regulated countries. This is likely to be a growing area of research over the next decade.

References

Döring G, Flume P, Heijerman H, et al. Treatment of lung infection in patients with cystic fibrosis: current and future strategies. *J Cyst Fibrosis* 2012;11:461–79.

Derichs N. Targeting a genetic defect: cystic fibrosis transmembrane conductance regulator modulators in cystic fibrosis. *Eur Respir Rev* 2013;22:58–65.

Goralski JL, Boucher RC, Button B. Osmolytes and ion transport modulators: new strategies for airway surface rehydration. *Curr Opin Pharmacol* 2010;10:294–9.

Griesenbach U, Alton EW. Progress in gene and cell therapy for cystic fibrosis lung disease. *Curr Pharm Des* 2012;18:642–62.

Kerem E, Konstan MW, De Boeck K, et al. Ataluren for the treatment of nonsense-mutation cystic fibrosis: a randomised, double-blind, placebo-controlled phase 3 trial. *Lancet Respiratory Medicine* 2014;2:539–47

Konstan MW, Döring G, Heltshe SL, et al. A randomized double blind, placebo controlled phase 2 trial of BIIL 284 BS (an LTB4 receptor antagonist) for the treatment of lung disease in children and adults with cystic fibrosis. *J Cyst Fibrosis* 2014;13(2):148–55.

Lands LC, Stanojevic S. Oral non-steroidal anti-inflammatory drug therapy for lung disease in cystic fibrosis. *Cochrane Database Syst Rev* 2013 Jun 13;6:CD001505.

Chapter 14

Pharmacy and the CF pharmacopoeia

Katrina Cox

Key points

- Once prescribed, medicines require monitoring for effectiveness and side effects; the CF specialist pharmacist is well placed to do this
- CF patients may exhibit differences in pharmacokinetics to subjects without CF. Drugs are often used at higher doses and for indications outside their licence
- The CF pharmacopoeia details important characteristics of medications commonly used in CF
- Allergies to medicines can pose a major challenge, but desensitization can be used in some to allow a previously contra-indicated antibiotic to be used

14.1 Introduction

As with all medicines, those for CF are administered with the intention of improving the health and quality of life of an individual, and the choice and dose is influenced by factors including:

- the desired outcome
- patient characteristics such as age, gender, weight, genotype, current clinical status
- other medical conditions
- other previous or current medication
- allergies
- patient preference

Once a medicine has been prescribed and administered to the patient, it must be monitored for efficacy, side effects, and continuing need. Patients, families, and other healthcare professionals involved in the care of the patient must also be offered information to allow the medicines to be used correctly. Collectively, this is known as providing 'pharmaceutical care' to patients.

14.2 Pharmacokinetics in CF

The pharmacokinetics of a drug describe the way the drug is absorbed into the body, the way it is distributed, metabolized, and then excreted from the body. These processes are affected by the intrinsic properties of the drug (such as the size of the molecule, lipophillicity), how the drug is administered to the patient (e.g. intravenously vs orally), and also by characteristics of the patient, such age, gender, existing medical conditions, other medicines, and clinical status.

CF can alter the pharmacokinetic properties of some drugs. For example, the volume of distribution of hydrophilic drugs such as aminoglycosides can be greater, so greater doses per kilogram of bodyweight may need to be used to achieve desired serum concentrations. Higher levels of gastric acid can reduce the absorption of some oral medications, whilst prolonged transit times through the gastrointestinal tract can have the opposite effect by enhancing absorption. Additionally, due to unclear mechanisms, some antibiotics such as β-lactams are eliminated more rapidly than in the non-CF population and CF patients may therefore require larger and more frequent doses.

14.3 **CF pharmacopoeia**

The CF pharmacopoeia aims to draw together information about the medicines used commonly within CF. It is not designed to be a comprehensive resource and clinicians may need to refer to the source literature for further information including the *British National Formulary* (BNF), the *BNF for Children*, the summary of product characteristics for individual medications, the *Renal Drug Handbook* or other national literature. Further information can be obtained from your CF specialist pharmacist.

The following abbreviations have been used:

OD—once daily

BD—twice daily

TDS—three times daily

QDS—four times daily

PRN—when required

14.3.1 **Antibiotics—oral and IV**

Antibiotics are used chronically as part of maintenance therapy (see Chapter 4) and as an acute treatment of respiratory infections (see Chapter 5). Indications given should be taken as indicative only. See Tables 14.1–14.33.

Table 14.1 Amikacin			
Treatment of early *Pseudomonas aeruginosa* infections not cleared by ciprofloxacin and colistimethate sodium, and of moderate and severe exacerbations of *Pseudomonas aeruginosa* infection. Treatment of *Mycobacterium abcessus*			
Aminoglycoside	Mode of action: bactericidal, inhibition of bacterial protein synthesis		
Adult dose:	**Paediatric dose:**	**Dosing in renal and hepatic impairment**	**Side effects**
IV 7.5 mg/kg BD or 15 mg/kg OD	IV 10 mg/kg (max 500 mg) TDS	Renal: reduce dose if GFR <50 ml/min Hepatic: no adjustment needed	Nephrotoxicity, ototoxicity
Counselling points/notes	Maintain adequate hydration, therapeutic drug monitoring required—refer to local guidelines. Dose according to ideal bodyweight in overweight or obese patients		

Table 14.2 Amoxicillin

Treatment of asymptomatic *Haemophilus influenzae* carriage or mild exacerbations (only use when a SENSITIVE STRAIN of *H.influenzae* has been identified and there has been no recent history of infection with *S.aureus*)

Aminopenicillin	Mode of action: bactericidal, inhibition of cell wall synthesis		
Adult dose:	**Paediatric dose:**	**Dosing in renal and hepatic impairment**	**Side effects**
Oral 500 mg TDS	Oral 1 month–1 year 125 mg TDS, 1 year–7 years 250 mg TDS, >7 years 500 mg TDS	Renal: reduce dose if GFR <10 ml/min Hepatic: no adjustment needed	GI disturbances, rash, rarely antibiotic-associated colitis
Counselling points/notes	None		

Table 14.3 Azithromycin

Long-term use in chronic *P.aeruginosa* infection

Macrolide	Mode of action: bacteriostatic, inhibition of bacterial protein synthesis		
Adult dose:	**Paediatric dose:**	**Dosing in renal and hepatic impairment**	**Side effects**
Oral 500 mg 3 × weekly, 250 mg 3 × weekly if <40 kg or 250 mg daily	Oral Over 6 months only. 10 mg/kg 3 × weekly if <15 kg 250 mg 3 × weekly if <40 kg 500 mg 3 × weekly if >40 kg	Renal: no dose adjustment necessary Hepatic: avoid in severe liver disease	Commonly, GI disturbances, less commonly, hepatotoxicity, QT elongation, reversible hearing loss, and tinnitus with prolonged use
Azithromycin			
Treatment of *Mycobacterium avium* complex			
Oral 500 mg daily	Oral 10 mg/kg daily (max 500 mg)	As above	As above
Counselling points/notes	Long term use is unlicensed Take on an empty stomach. Avoid in severe liver disease		

Table 14.4 Aztreonam

Treatment of *P.aeruginosa* exacerbations if unable to use first-line agents

Monocyclic β-lactam (monolactam)	Mode of action: bactericidal, inhibition of bacterial cell wall synthesis		
Adult dose:	**Paediatric dose:**	**Dosing in renal and hepatic impairment**	**Side effects**
IV 2 g TDS—QDS (3 g TDS can also be used off licence)	IV 1 month–2 years 30 mg/kg (max 2 g) TDS-QDS, 2 years–12 years 50 mg/kg (max 2 g) TDS—QDS, >12 years 2 g TDS—QDS	Renal: reduce dose if GFR <30 ml/min Hepatic: use with caution and monitor liver function	GI bleeding, rarely antibiotic-associated colitis, GI disturbances, jaundice, hepatitis, blood disorders
Counselling points/notes	No gram-positive activity, so use with an aminoglycoside		

Table 14.5 Cefaclor

Treatment of asymptomatic *H.influenzae* carriage or mild exacerbations

Second-generation cephalosporin	Mode of action: bactericidal, inhibition of bacterial cell wall synthesis		
Adult dose:	**Paediatric dose:**	**Dosing in renal and hepatic impairment**	**Side effects**
Oral 500 mg TDS	Oral 1 month–1 year 125 mg TDS, 1–7 years 250 mg TDS, > 7 years 500 mg TDS	Renal: reduce dose if GFR <10 ml/min Hepatic: no adjustment needed	Commonly GI disturbances, hypersensitivity reactions such as rashes, disturbances in LFTs, transient hepatitis and cholestatic jaundice, blood disorders
Counselling points/notes	None		

Table 14.6 Cefixime

Treatment of asymptomatic *H.influenzae* carriage or mild exacerbations

Third-generation cephalosporin	Mode of action: bactericidal, inhibition of bacterial cell wall synthesis		
Adult dose:	**Paediatric dose:**	**Dosing in renal and hepatic impairment**	**Side effects**
Oral 400 mg OD	Oral 6 months–1 year 75 mg OD, 1–5 years 100 mg OD, 5–10 years 200 mg OD, >10 years 400 mg OD	Renal: reduce dose if GFR <10 ml/min Hepatic: No adjustment needed	Commonly GI disturbances, hypersensitivity reactions such as rashes, disturbances in LFTs, transient hepatitis, and cholestatic jaundice
Counselling points/notes	None		

Table 14.7 Cefotaxime

Treatment of severe *H. influenzae* exacerbations

Third-generation cephalosporin	Mode of action: bactericidal, inhibition of bacterial cell wall synthesis			
Adult dose:	**Paediatric dose:**	**Dosing in renal and hepatic impairment**	**Side effects**	
IV 2 g TDS, dose can be increased if necessary to 12 g in 24 hours	IV 1 month–18 years 50 mg/kg TDS—QDS (max 12 g in 24 hours)	Renal: reduce dose if GFR <10ml/min Hepatic: no adjustment needed	Commonly GI disturbances, hypersensitivity reactions such as rashes, disturbances in LFTs, transient hepatitis and cholestatic jaundice, blood disorders	
Counselling points/notes	None			

Table 14.8 Cefoxitin

Treatment of *Mycobacterium abcessus*

Semisynthetic β-lactam	Mode of action: bactericidal, inhibition of bacterial cell wall synthesis		
Adult dose:	**Paediatric dose:**	**Dosing in renal and hepatic impairment**	**Side effects**
IV 2–3 g QDS	IV 40 mg/kg (max 3000 mg) QDS	Renal: reduce dose if GFR <50 ml/min Hepatic: no adjustment needed	GI disturbances, hypersensitivity reactions
Counselling points/notes	Unlicensed in the UK, interferes with laboratory creatinine results		

Table 14.9 Ceftazidime

Treatment of *P.aeruginosa* and *B.cepacia* exacerbation

Third-generation cephalosporin	Mode of action: bactericidal, inhibition of bacterial cell wall synthesis		
Adult dose:	**Paediatric dose:**	**Dosing in renal and hepatic impairment**	**Side effects**
IV 2–3 g TDS Doses of up to 3 g QDS can be used off licence	IV 1 month–18 years 50 mg/kg (max 3 g) TDS	Renal: reduce dose if GFR <50 ml/min Hepatic: caution in severe hepatic impairment	Commonly GI disturbances, hypersensitivity reactions such as rashes, rarely antibiotic-associated colitis
Counselling points/notes	None		

Table 14.10 Chloramphenicol

Treatment of *H.influenzae*, *P.aeruginosa*, and *B.cepacia* exacerbation where first line antibiotics are unsuitable for use

Synthetic antibiotic, unique in nature	Mode of action: bacteriostatic, inhibits bacterial protein synthesis		
Adult dose:	**Paediatric dose:**	**Dosing in renal and hepatic impairment**	**Side effects**
Oral (less severe infections) IV (more severe infections) 12.5–25 mg/kg QDS	Oral (less severe infections) IV (more severe infections) 12.5–25 mg/kg QDS	Renal: no dose adjustment needed, but avoid if possible in severe impairment Hepatic: avoid in hepatic impairment	Blood disorders including reversible and irreversible aplastic anaemias, peripheral and optic neuritis
Counselling points/notes	Should only be used when other options have been exhausted. Patient should receive alternate day FBC monitoring Also active against *S.aureus*		

Table 14.11 Ciprofloxacin

Treatment of *P.aeruginosa*, first isolates and chronically colonized patients with a mild exacerbation

Quinolone	Mode of action: bactericidal, inhibition of bacterial metabolism		
Adult dose:	**Paediatric dose:**	**Dosing in renal and hepatic impairment**	**Side effects**
Oral 750 mg BD Doses of up to 1 g BD used (off licence)	Oral 1 month–5 years 15 mg/kg BD, 5 years–18 years 20 mg/kg (max 750 mg) BD	Renal: reduce dose if GFR <20 ml/min Hepatic: no adjustment needed	Commonly GI disturbances, photosensitivity, rarely convulsions (especially if co-administered with NSAIDs or theophylline)
Ciprofloxacin			
Treatment of *P.aeruginosa* exacerbation when first-line IV treatments are unsuitable			
IV 400 mg BD-TDS	IV Neonate 10 mg/kg BD, 1 month–18 years 10 mg/kg BD-TDS, (max 400 mg TDS)	As above	As above
Counselling points/notes	Quinolones cause arthropathy in the weight-bearing joints of immature *animals* and are therefore generally not recommended in children and growing adolescents. However, the significance of this effect in humans is uncertain and short-term use based upon need may be justified in children. Avoid direct sunlight and the use of sun beds. Keep at least 2 hours apart from milk, indigestion remedies, iron, and zinc		

Table 14.12 Clarithromycin

IV: Treatment of *Mycobacterium abcessus*

Oral: Treatment of *Mycobacterium avium* complex and atypical infection such as *Mycoplasma* or non-tuberculous mycobacteria

Macrolide	Mode of action: bactericidal, inhibition of bacterial protein synthesis		
Adult dose:	**Paediatric dose:**	**Dosing in renal and hepatic impairment**	**Side effects**
Oral / IV 500 mg BD	Oral / IV <12 years or <30 kg 7.5 mg/kg BD (max 500 mg per dose), >12 years or >30 kg	Renal: reduce dose if GFR <30 ml/min Hepatic: caution, can cause further dysfunction or jaundice	Commonly GI disturbances, less commonly hepatotoxicity, QT elongation, rarely tinnitus
Counselling points/notes	Interactions with other medicines common		

Table 14.13 Clindamycin

Treatment of asymptomatic *Staphylococcus aureus* isolates or minor exacerbations

Lincosamide	Mode of action: bacteriostatic, inhibition of bacterial protein synthesis		
Adult dose:	**Paediatric dose:**	**Dosing in renal and hepatic impairment**	**Side effects**
Oral 600 mg QDS (450 mg is maximum licensed dose)	Oral 1month–18 years 5–7 mg/ kg (max 600 mg) QDS (450 mg is maximum licensed dose)	Renal: no dose reduction required Hepatic: no adjustment needed	Diarrhoea, antibiotic associated colitis, taste disturbances, jaundice, blood dyscrasis
Counselling points/notes	Patients should discontinue immediately and seek medical advice if diarrhoea develops Monitor LFTs and renal function if treatment exceeds 10 days		

Table 14.14 Co-amoxiclav (amoxicillin and clavulanic acid)

Treatment of asymptomatic *Haemophilus influenzae* carriage or mild exacerbations

Aminopenicillin plus β-lactamase inhibitor	Mode of action: bactericidal, inhibition of cell wall synthesis		
Adult dose:	**Paediatric dose:**	**Dosing in renal and hepatic impairment**	**Side effects**
Oral 625 mg TDS	Oral 1 month–1 year 0.5ml/kg of the 125/31 suspension TDS, 1–6 years 5 ml of the 250/62 suspension TDS, 6 – 12 years 10 ml of the 250/62 suspension TDS, >12 years 625 mg TDS	Renal: reduce dose if GFR <10 ml/min Hepatic: monitor LFTs in existing impairment	GI disturbances, rashes, hepatitis, cholestatic jaundice, rarely antibiotic associated colitis
Counselling points/ notes	Contains a penicillin, monitor liver function in existing liver disease. Cholestatic jaundice possibly associated with clavulanic acid		

Table 14.15 Colistimethate sodium

Treatment of *P.aeruginosa* exacerbation when first line IV treatments are unsuitable

Polymyxin	Mode of action: bactericidal, acts like a cationic surfactant. Binds to susceptible bacterial cytoplasmic membranes, alters its osmotic properties, and causes leakage of intracellular contents		
Adult dose:	**Paediatric dose:**	**Dosing in renal and hepatic impairment**	**Side effects**
IV 2 MU (megaunits) TDS	IV <60 kg 0.25 MU/kg TDS >60 kg 2MU TDS	Renal: use with caution if GFR <50 ml/min, reduce dose if GFR <20 ml/min Hepatic: no adjustment needed	Neurotoxicity with excessive doses, nephrotoxicity, rash
Counselling points/notes	Monitor renal function, use with caution with other nephrotoxic medicines		

Table 14.16 Co-trimoxazole (sulfamethoxazole and trimethoprim)

Treatment of *B.cepacia* and *Stenotrophomonas maltophilia* infections

Sulfamethoxazole: sulfonamide Trimethoprim: synthetic folate-antagonist	Mode of action: sulfamethoxazole: bacteriostatic, inhibits essential bacterial enzyme Trimethoprim: synthetic folate-antagonist		
Adult dose:	**Paediatric dose:**	**Dosing in renal and hepatic impairment**	**Side effects**
Oral 960 mg BD IV 960 mg BD	Oral 6 wks–6 m 120 mg BD, 6m–6 years 240 mg BD, 6–12 years 480 mg BD, >12 years 960 mg BD IV: 6 m–6 years 240 mg BD, 6–12 years 480 mg BD, >12 years 960 mg BD	Renal: reduce dose if GFR <30 ml/min Hepatic: avoid in severe liver disease	GI disturbances, hyperkalaemia, rarely Stevens–Johnson syndrome, blood dyscrasias
Counselling points/notes	Avoid in G6PD deficiency		

Table 14.17 Doxycycline

Treatment of asymptomatic *Haemophilus influenzae* and *B.cepacia* carriage or mild exacerbations

Tetracycline	Mode of action: bacteriostatic, inhibition of bacterial protein synthesis		
Adult dose:	**Paediatric dose:**	**Dosing in renal and hepatic impairment**	**Side effects**
Oral 200 mg first day, 100–200 mg daily thereafter	Oral Contra-indicated <12 years. >12 years 200 mg first day, 100–200 mg daily thereafter	Renal: no dose reduction required Hepatic: avoid or use with caution in patients with liver impairment	GI disturbances, occasionally antibiotic associated colitis, dysphagia, oesophageal irritation, hepatotoxicity, blood disorders, hypersensitivity reactions
Counselling points/notes	Swallow whole with a glass of water. Keep at least 2 hours apart from milk, indigestion remedies, iron, and zinc. Avoid direct sunlight and the use of sunbeds		

Table 14.18 Ethambutol

Treatment of *Mycobacterium avium* complex and atypical infection such as *Mycoplasma* and non-tuberculous mycobacteria

Antituberculosis	Mode of action: not clear, possibly diffuses into susceptible organism and suppresses replication by interfering with RNA synthesis		
Adult dose:	**Paediatric dose:**	**Dosing in renal and hepatic impairment**	**Side effects**
Oral 15 mg/kg (max 1.5 g) OD	Oral 15 mg/kg (max 1.5 g) OD (caution in <5 years due to inability to report visual changes—see counselling points/notes)	Renal: reduce dose if GFR <20 ml/min Hepatic: no dose adjustment is needed	Optic neuritis, red/green colour blindness, peripheral neuritis, rarely rash, pruritus, urticaria, thrombocytopenia
Counselling points/notes	Patients should be advised to discontinue therapy immediately if they develop deterioration in vision and promptly seek further advice		

Table 14.19 Flucloxacillin

See below for indications

Penicillinase resistant penicillin	Mode of action: bactericidal, inhibition of cell wall synthesis		
Adult dose:	**Paediatric dose:**	**Dosing in renal and hepatic impairment**	**Side effects**
Continuous anti-staphylococcal therapy: Oral Only with recurrent MSSA growth, 50 mg/kg BD	Oral Birth–3 years 125 mg BD, >3 years, only with recurrent MSSA growth, 50mg/kg BD	Renal: reduce dose if GFR <10 ml/min Hepatic: use with caution in patients with a history of hepatic dysfunction	Hypersensitivity reactions, GI disturbances, rarely CNS toxicity including convulsions, very rarely cholestatic jaundice and hepatitis
Treatment of asymptomatic *Staphylococcus aureus* isolates or minor exacerbations Oral 1–2 g QDS	Oral <18 years 25mg/kg QDS	As above	As above
Treatment of more severe exacerbations caused by *Staphylococcus aureus* IV 2–3 g QDS	IV 1 month–18 years 50 mg/kg QDS	As above	As above
Counselling points/ notes	Take on an empty stomach		

Table 14.20 Fosfomycin

Treatment of exacerbation with Gram-positive or Gram-negative bacteria including *S.aureus*, *H.influenzae* and *P.aeruginosa* when first line IV treatments are unsuitable

Phosphonic acid	Mode of action: Bactericidal, inhibition of bacterial cell wall synthesis		
Adult dose:	**Paediatric dose:**	**Dosing in renal and hepatic impairment**	**Side effects**
IV 4 g TDS—QDS (up to 24 g/day have been used in severe infections)	IV Up to 4 weeks 200mg/ kg in three divided doses 1–12 months (up to 10kg) 200–300mg/kg in three divided doses 1–12 years (up to 40kg) 200–400mg/kg in 3–4 divided doses	Renal: Reduce dose when GFR <40ml/min Hepatic: No Dose adjustment required	GI side effects, transient increases in levels of aminotransferases, headache, visual disturbances, skin rashes
Counselling points/notes	None		

Table 14.21 Linezolid

Treatment of refractory MRSA. Also *Mycobacterium abcessus* (when first line agents are unsuitable). Also treatment of severe exacerbations of *Staphylococcus aureus*

Oxazolidinone	Mode of action: bacteriostatic, inhibition of ribosomal protein synthesis		
Adult dose:	**Paediatric dose:**	**Dosing in renal and hepatic impairment**	**Side effects**
IV and Oral 600 mg BD	IV and Oral 1 month–12 years 10 mg/kg (max 600 mg) TDS, >12 years 600 mg BD	Renal: if GFR <10 ml/ min, increase frequency of platelet monitoring and reduce dose to OD if they fall Hepatic: only use in severe impairment if potential benefit outweighs the risk	GI disturbances, including antibiotic associated colitis, taste disturbances, headache. Also blood disorders including thrombocytopenia, anaemia, leucopenia, and pancytopenia. Risk of optic neuropathy, especially if used for >28 days. See BNF for further information
Counselling points/notes	There is little advantage to using the IV preparation due to high bioavailability. Linezolid is a reversible, non-selective monoamine oxidase inhibitor (MAOI). Patients should avoid consuming large amounts of tyramine-rich foods. In addition, linezolid should not be given within 2 weeks of using another MAOI. Use with caution and avoid if possible in those receiving SSRIs, 5HT agonists ('triptans'), tricyclic antidepressants, sympathomimetics, dopaminergics, buspirone, pethidine, and possibly other opioid analgesics Monitor FBC at least weekly		

Table 14.22 Minocycline

Treatment of *Stenotrophomonas maltophilia* and *Achromobacter xylosoxidans* exacerbation where first line choices are unsuitable

Tetracycline	Mode of action: bacteriostatic, inhibition of bacterial protein synthesis		
Adult dose:	**Paediatric dose:**	**Dosing in renal and hepatic impairment**	**Side effects**
Oral 100 mg BD	Oral Unlicensed for <12 years 12–18 years 100 mg BD	Renal: no dose reduction required Hepatic: avoid or use with caution in hepatic impairment	GI disturbances, dizziness and vertigo, dysphagia, photosensitivity
Counselling points/notes	Unlicensed in children under 12 years. Tablets or capsules should be swallowed whole with plenty of fluid while sitting or standing Use with caution in patients receiving other potentially hepatotoxic drugs		

Table 14.23 Meropenem

Treatment of *P.aeruginosa*, *B.cepacia*, *M.abcessus*, and *Achromobacter xylosoxidans* exacerbation

Carbapenem	Mode of action: bactericidal, inhibition of bacterial cell wall synthesis		
Adult dose:	**Paediatric dose:**	**Dosing in renal and hepatic impairment**	**Side effects**
IV 1–2 g TDS	IV 4–18 years <50 kg 25–40 mg/kg (max 2g) TDS 4–18 years >50 kg 1–2 g TDS	Renal: reduce dose if GFR <50 ml/min Hepatic: monitor liver function in patients with existing impairment	GI disturbances, derangements in LFTs, headache, haematological abnormalities
Counselling points/notes	Can be used in children >1 month if necessary		

Table 14.24 Piperacillin/Tazobactam

Treatment of *P.aeruginosa*, *B.cepacia*, and *Achromobacter xylosoxidans* exacerbations when first-line antibiotics not suitable

Piperacillin: A semi-synthetic extended-spectrum ureidopenicillin. Tazobactam: a β-lactamase inhibitor	Mode of action: bactericidal, inhibition of cell wall synthesis		
Adult dose:	**Paediatric dose:**	**Dosing in renal and hepatic impairment**	**Side effects**
IV 4.5g TDS—QDS	IV <12 years 90 mg/kg (max 4.5 g) TDS—QDS >12 years 4.5 g TDS—QDS	Renal: reduce dose if GFR <20 ml/min Hepatic: no dose adjustment required	Hypersensitivity reactions, rarely CNS toxicity including convulsions, blood dyscrasias
Counselling points/notes	Due to risk of blood dyscrasias, limit courses to 14 days		

Table 14.25 Rifampicin

Other class	Mode of action: bactericidal, inhibition of DNA-dependent RNA polymerase activity in susceptible cells		
Adult dose:	**Paediatric dose:**	**Dosing in renal and hepatic impairment**	**Side effects**
As part of prolonged combination therapy for *Mycobacterium avium* complex eradication Oral <50 kg 450 mg OD, >50 kg 600 mg OD	Oral 10 mg/kg OD (not exceeding adult dose)	Renal: consider dose reduction if GFR<10 ml/min Hepatic: monitor liver function in patients with existing impairment	GI disturbances, headache, drowsiness, hepatic dysfunction
Treatment of asymptomatic *S. aureus* isolates or minor exacerbations and as part of combination therapy for MRSA eradication Oral 600 mg BD	Oral 1 month–1 year 5–10 mg/kg BD, 1–18 years 10 mg/kg (max 450 mg <50 kg and max 600 mg >50 kg) BD	As above	As above
Counselling points/notes	Take on an empty stomach. Turns bodily fluids orange/red; avoid wearing contact lenses. Patients should know to reports signs of hepatic dysfunction (persistent nausea, vomiting, malaise or jaundice). Potent liver enzyme inducer with many interactions with other medicines including hormonal contraceptives for up to 6 weeks		

Table 14.26 Sodium fusidate (Fusidic acid)

Treatment of *S.aureus* colonisation or exacerbation and as part of combination therapy for MRSA eradication

Steroidal antibiotic	Mode of action: bactiostatic and bactericidal, inhibition of bacterial protein synthesis		
Adult dose:	**Paediatric dose:**	**Dosing in renal and hepatic impairment**	**Side effects**
Oral Dose as fusidic acid for the **liquid preparation**: 750 mg TDS Dose as fusidate for **the tablet formulation**: 500 mg TDS	Oral Doses as fusidic acid for the **liquid preparation:** 1 month–1 year 15 mg/kg TDS, 1–5 years 250 mg TDS, 5–12 years 500 mg TDS, >12 years 750 mg TDS	Renal: no dose adjustment required Hepatic: avoid in severe liver disease.	GI disturbances, drowsiness, dizziness, hepatotoxicity
Counselling points/notes	Doses quoted as fusidic acid and as fusidate, take care when selecting dose. Monitor LFTs with prolonged courses		

Table 14.27 Teicoplanin

Treatment of MRSA exacerbation, treatment of severe exacerbations of *S.aureus*

Glycopeptide	Mode of action: bactericidal, inhibits bacterial cell wall synthesis		
Adult dose:	**Paediatric dose:**	**Dosing in renal and hepatic impairment**	**Side effects**
IV 10 mg/kg (max 400 mg) BD on day 1, then 10 mg/kg (max licensed dose 400 mg, but local policies may advocate higher doses) OD thereafter	IV 1 month–18 years 10 mg/kg (max 400 mg) BD on day 1, then 10 mg/kg (max 400 mg) OD thereafter	Renal: reduce dose if GFR <20 ml/min Hepatic: no dose adjustment required	Rash, GI disturbances, blood disorders, tinnitus, renal dysfunction
Counselling points/notes	Levels can be checked to optimize therapy. Trough levels should be between 20 mg/l and 60 mg/l. Use with caution in patients with a history of vancomycin sensitivity		

Table 14.28 Temocillin

Treatment of *B.cepacia* exacerbation

Semi-synthetic β-lactam	Mode of action: bactericidal, inhibition of bacterial cell wall synthesis		
Adult dose:	**Paediatric dose:**	**Dosing in renal and hepatic impairment**	**Side effects**
>45 kg 1–2 g BD	IV >12 years and >45 kg 1–2 g BD (Off licence for <18 years)	Renal: reduce dose if GFR <30 ml/min Hepatic: no dose adjustment required	Hypersensitivity reactions, rarely CNS toxicity including convulsions
Counselling points/notes	Not active against *P.aeruginosa*		

Table 14.29 Tigecycline

Treatment of *Stenotrophomonas maltophilia* exacerbation and *M.abcessus* exacerbation when first-line antibiotics are unsuitable

Glycylcycline (related to the tetracyclines)	Mode of action: bacteriostatic, inhibition of bacterial protein synthesis		
Adult dose:	**Paediatric dose:**	**Dosing in renal and hepatic impairment**	**Side effects**
IV 100 mg initial dose, then 50 mg BD	IV >12 years 50 mg BD (Off licence <18 years)	Renal: no dose reduction required Hepatic: initially 100 mg then 25 mg every 12 hours in severe impairment	GI disturbances, dizziness, headache, prolonged prothrombin time
Counselling points/notes	Can cause hypoglycaemia		

Table 14.30 Tobramycin

Pulmonary exacerbation regardless of sputum microbiology

Aminoglycoside	Mode of action: bactericidal, inhibition of protein synthesis		
Adult dose:	**Paediatric dose:**	**Dosing in renal and hepatic impairment**	**Side effects**
IV 10 mg/kg OD (max 660 mg)	IV 10mg/kg OD (max 660 mg)	Renal: reduce if GFR <50 ml/min. Adjust according to trough levels Hepatic: no dose adjustment required	Nephrotoxicity and ototoxicity
Counselling points/notes	Trough levels should be taken before the second dose and then weekly if patient is stable. A level of <1 mg/l should be achieved. Dose or dose interval can be adjusted if required to achieve these levels. Repeated courses increase risk of nephro- and ototoxicity. Dose according to ideal body weight if patient is overweight or obese		

Table 14.31 Ticarcillin/clavulanic acid

Treatment of *P.aeruginosa* exacerbation and in treatment of *S.maltophilia* when first line antibiotics are unsuitable

Ticarcillin: extended-spectrum carboxypenicillin. Clavulanic acid: β-lactamase inhibitor	Mode of action: bactericidal, inhibition of bacterial cell wall synthesis		
Adult dose:	**Paediatric dose:**	**Dosing in renal and hepatic impairment**	**Side effects**
IV 3.2 g TDS—QDS	IV 1 month–18 years 80–100 mg/kg (max 3.2 g) TDS—QDS	Renal: reduce dose if GFR <50 ml/min Hepatic: avoid in severe impairment	Hypersensitivity reactions, rarely CNS toxicity including convulsions, GI disturbances, coagulation disorders
Counselling points/notes	Cholestatic jaundice possibly associated with clavulanic acid		

Table 14.32 Trimethoprim

Treatment of *Burkholderia cepacia* infections. As part of combination therapy for MRSA eradication

Dihydrofolate reductase inhibitor	Mode of action: both bactiostatic and bactericidal, inhibits bacterial amino acid synthesis		
Adult dose:	**Paediatric dose:**	**Dosing in renal and hepatic impairment**	**Side effects**
Oral 200 mg BD	Oral 6 months–12 years 4 mg/kg (max 200mg) BD	Renal: no dose reduction required Hepatic: no dose adjustment required	GI disturbances, rashes, hyperkalaemia, blood dyscrasias
Counselling points/notes	On long-term treatment, patients should be told how to recognize signs of blood disorders and advised to seek immediate medical attention if symptoms such as fever, sore throat, rash, mouth ulcers, purpura, bruising, or bleeding develop		

Table 14.33 Vancomycin

Treatment of MRSA exacerbation and severe *S.aureus* exacerbations			
Glycopeptide	Mode of action: bactericidal, inhibits bacterial cell wall synthesis		
Adult dose:	**Paediatric dose:**	**Dosing in renal and hepatic impairment**	**Side effects**
IV 1 g BD (dose adjusted according to levels, local policies may advocate higher doses)	IV 1 month–18 years 15 mg/kg TDS (dose adjusted according to levels	Renal: reduces dose if GFR <20 ml/min Hepatic: no dose adjustment required	Nephrotoxicity, ototoxicity, blood disorders including neutropenia (usually after one week or a cumulative dose of 25 g)
Counselling points/notes	Trough and peak levels are checked to prevent accumulation and ensure therapeutic peak concentrations are reached. Refer to local policies. Patients should be told how to recognise signs of blood disorders, e.g. fever, sore throat, rash, mouth ulcers, purpura, bruising, or bleeding Can cause red man syndrome if administered too rapidly		

14.3.2 **Antibiotics—nebulized and inhaled**

Nebulized and inhaled antibiotics deliver medication directly to the lungs. Reference should be made to national funding arrangements before prescribing. See Tables 14.34–14.39.

Table 14.34 Amikacin (unlicensed)

Treatment or suppression of chronic infection with *Mycobacterium abscessus*			
Administration: via a nebulizer attached to an air/oxygen supply. Vials made up to 4 ml using sodium chloride 0.9%			
Adult dose:	**Paediatric dose:**	**Contra-indications and cautions**	**Side effects**
500 mg BD	<12 years 250 mg BD, >12 years 500 mg BD	Contra-indications: concurrent use of IV aminoglycosides, hypersensitivity to any aminoglycoside Cautions: existing renal impairment, haemoptysis	Nephro- and oto-toxicity, bronchospasm, cough
Counselling points/notes	Unlicensed. Requires a challenge test with measures of lung function pre and post dose under supervision to ensure tolerability. Monitor renal function and hearing before treatment and then annually		

Table 14.35 Aztreonam (brand name Cayston®)

Suppression of chronic infection with *Pseudomonas aeruginosa*

Administration: nebulized via an eBase® Controller or an eFlow® Rapid Control Unit used with the Altera Nebuliser Handset® and Altera Aerosol Head®

Adult dose:	Paediatric dose:	Contra-indications and cautions	Side effects
75 mg TDS alternate months	>6 years 75 mg TDS alternate months	Contra-indications: hypersensitivity to aztreonam Cautions: hypersensitivity to beta-lactams, haemoptysis	Wheezing, bronchospasm, cough, haemoptysis, pyrexia, arthralgia, rash, rhinorrhoea, pharyngolaryngeal pain
Counselling points/notes	Requires a challenge test with measures of lung function pre and post dose under supervision to ensure tolerability. Other inhaled or nebulized medication should be administered prior to aztreonam		

Table 14.36 Colistimethate sodium

Treatment or suppression of chronic infection with *Pseudomonas aeruginosa*

Adult dose:	Paediatric dose:	Contra-indications and cautions	Side effects
Brand name **Colomycin®**: administration via a nebulizer attached to an air/oxygen supply. Vials dissolved in 2–4 ml water for injection or sodium chloride 0.9%			
1–2 million units BD	1 month – 2 years, 0.5–1 million units BD—TDS, >2 years 1–2 million units BD—TDS	Contra-indications: myasthenia gravis, hypersensitivity to colistimethate sodium Cautions: haemoptysis	Sore throat, sore mouth, taste disturbances, nausea, vomiting, cough, bronchospasm, dysphonia, thirst, hypersalivation
Brand name **Promixin®**: administration via various nebulizer systems. Diluent is either water for injection or sodium chloride 0.9%			
1–2 million IU 2 or 3 times daily	>2 years 1–2 million IU 2 or 3 times daily	As above	As above
Brand name **Colobreathe®**: administration by inhalation via a Turbospin powder inhaler®			
1.66 MU (approximately equivalent to 125 mg) BD	>6 years 1.66 MU (approximately equivalent to 125 mg) BD	As above	As above
Counselling points/notes	All 3 delivery systems require a challenge test with measures of lung function pre and post dose under supervision to ensure tolerability before initiation. Other inhaled or nebulized medication should be administered prior to colistimethate sodium		

Table 14.37 Meropenem (unlicensed)

Treatment or suppression of chronic infection with *Pseudomonas aeruginosa*, if the use of other inhaled/nebulized anti pseudomonals is not suitable

Administration: via a nebulizer attached to an air/oxygen supply. 500 mg vials reconstituted with 10 ml water for injection and 5 ml nebulized. Remaining solution must be discarded

Adult dose:	Paediatric dose:	Contra-indications and cautions	Side effects
250 mg BD	250 mg BD	Contra-indications: concurrent use of IV meropenem, hypersensitivity to meropenem Cautions: hypersensitvity to beta-lactams, haemoptysis	Bronchospasm, cough, staining of teeth
Counselling points/notes	Unlicensed. Requires a challenge test with measures of lung function pre and post dose under supervision to ensure tolerability		

Table 14.38 Tobramycin

Treatment or suppression of chronic infection with *Pseudomonas aeruginosa*

Adult dose:	Paediatric dose:	Contra-indications and cautions	Side effects
Administration: nebulized via a PARI LC PLUS® reusable nebulizer with a suitable compressor			
Brand name **TOBI®**: 300 mg/5ml BD alternate months Brand name **Bramitob®**: 300 mg/4ml BD alternate months	Brand name **TOBI®**: >6 years 300 mg/5ml BD alternate months Brand name **Bramitob®**: 300 mg/4ml BD alternate months	Contra-indications: hypersensitivity to any aminoglycoside Cautions: haemoptysis, existing renal impairment	Bronchospasm, cough
Administration: inhaled via the **TOBI Podhaler**			
Contents of 4 × 28 mg capsules BD alternate months	>6 years Contents of 4 × 28mg capsules BD alternate months	As above	As above
Counselling points/notes	All three require a challenge test with measures of lung function pre and post dose under supervision to ensure tolerability. Monitor renal function and hearing before treatment and then annually		

Table 14.39 Vancomycin (unlicensed)

Eradication treatment of chronic infection with MRSA

Administration: via a nebulizer attached to an air/oxygen supply. 500 mg vial reconstituted with 10 ml water for injection and 4 ml (200 mg) or 5 ml (250 mg) withdrawn

Adult dose:	Paediatric dose:	Contra-indications and cautions	Side effects
200–250 mg QDS	4 mg/kg (max 250 mg) BD-QDS	Contra-indications: concurrent use of IV amino-glycosides, hypersensitivity to vancomycin or teicoplanin Cautions: existing renal impairment, haemoptysis	Nephro- and ototoxicity, bronchospasm cough
Counselling points/notes	Unlicensed. Requires a challenge test with measures of lung function pre and post dose under supervision to ensure tolerability. Monitor renal function and hearing before treatment and then annually Make up to 4 ml using sodium chloride 0.9% or sterile water		

14.3.3 **Antifungals**

Lung infections with fungi can occur in CF, or more commonly allergic bronchopulmonary aspergillosis (ABPA) may require suppression therapy (see Chapter 4). See Tables 14.40–14.42.

Table 14.40 Amphotericin (unlicensed)

Treatment of ABPA

Administration: 50 mg Fungizone® (liposomal amphotericin B) vial reconstituted with 12 ml water for injection and 6 ml (25 mg) withdrawn to nebulize

Adult dose:	Paediatric dose:	Contra-indications and cautions	Side effects
Nebulized: 25 mg BD	Nebulized: 25 mg BD	Contra-indications: hypersensitivity to amphotericin Cautions: haemoptysis	Bronchospasm, cough
Counselling points/notes	Unlicensed. Requires a challenge test with measures of lung function pre and post dose under supervision to ensure tolerability. Monitor renal function and hearing before treatment, and then annually		

Table 14.41 Itraconazole

Treatment of ABPA

Adult dose:	Paediatric dose:	Dosing in renal and hepatic impairment	Side effects
Oral: 200 mg BD Dose adjusted to levels	Oral: 1 month – 18 years 5 mg/kg daily	Renal: no dose reduction required Hepatic: avoid in those with existing hepatic impairment	Potentially life-threatening heptox-icity occurs very rarely, discontinue treatment if signs of hepatitis Monitor liver function in those receiving therapy for longer than 1 month, in those receiving other potentially hepatotoxic drugs Many interactions, including poten-tiation of some inhaled steroids
Counselling points/ notes	Many interactions, check existing medication before commencing. Patients should be told how to recognize signs of liver disorder and advised to seek prompt medical attention if symptoms such as ano-rexia, nausea, vomiting, fatigue, abdominal pain, or dark urine develop. Requires TDM, levels can be taken at any time and should be within the range of 5–15 mg/l Liquid—take on an empty stomach Capsules—take with or after food, preferably with an acidic drink Caution: avoid in patients with a history of heart failure, or in patients at a high risk of heart disease Contra-indicated in acute porphyria		

Table 14.42 Voriconazole

Treatment of ABPA

Adult dose:	Paediatric dose:	Dosing in renal and hepatic impairment	Side effects
Oral >40 kg, 400 mg BD for 2 doses then 200 mg BD, increased if neces-sary to 300 mg BD, >18 years and <40 kg, 200 mg BD for 2 doses then 100 mg BD, increased if neces-sary to 150 mg BD	Oral <12 years 200 mg BD >12 years and <40 kg 200 mg BD for 1 day, then 100 mg BD >12 years and >40 kg 400 mg BD for 1 day, then 200 mg BD	Renal: no dose reduc-tion required Hepatic: avoid in those with existing hepatic impairment	GI disturbances, oedema, hypoten-sion, blood disorders, uncommonly hepatitis, cholestasis, and ful-minant hepatic failure (usually in first 10 days)
Counselling points/ notes	Monitor liver function before and during treatment. Take with or after food. Voriconazole has a moderate influence on the ability to drive and use machines. It may cause transient and reversible changes to vision, including blurring, altered/enhanced visual perception, and/or photo-phobia. Patients must avoid potentially hazardous tasks, such as driving or operating machinery while experiencing these symptoms. Many inter-actions, check existing medication before commencing. Contra-indicated in acute porphyria		

14.3.4 **Mucolytics**

The objective of these is to mobilize lower respiratory tract secretions and relieve mucus impaction in the airways. See Tables 14.43–14.45.

Table 14.43 Recombinant human dnase, dornase alfa (brand name Pulmozyme®)

Administration: via a nebulizer attached to an air/oxygen supply

Adult dose:	Paediatric dose:	Contra-indications and cautions	Side effects
2.5 mg OD, if >21 years, can be increased to BD	>5 years 2.5 mg OD	Contra-indications: hypersensitivity to dornase alfa or any of the excipients Cautions: haemoptysis	Rarely dyspepsia, chest pain, dysphonia, dyspnoea, pharyngitis, laryngitis, pyrexia, conjunctivitis, rhinitis, rash, urticaria
Counselling points/notes	Requires a challenge test with measures of lung function pre and post dose under supervision to ensure tolerability Only licensed for patients with a FVC >40%, although commonly used in patients with lower FVC %		

Table 14.44 Hypertonic saline solutions (7% brand name Nebusal®; 3% or 6% brand name Mucoclear®)

Administration: via a nebulizer attached to an air/oxygen supply

Adult dose:	Paediatric dose:	Contra-indications and cautions	Side effects
1–4 ml OD	1–4 ml OD	Contra-indications: hypersensitivity to hypertonic saline solutions Cautions: haemoptysis	Temporary irritation, such as coughing, hoarseness, or reversible bronchoconstriction
Counselling points/notes	Requires a challenge test with measures of lung function pre and post dose under supervision to ensure tolerability		

Table 14.45 Mannitol (Bronchitol®)

Administration: Contents of 10 × 40 mg capsules inhaled via the inhaler device provided by the manufacturer

Adult dose:	Paediatric dose:	Contra-indications and cautions	Side effects
400 mg BD	Not licensed <18 years	Contra-indications: hypersensitivity to mannitol Cautions: haemoptysis	Vomiting, cough, wheezing, haemoptysis, throat irritation, pharyngolaryngeal pain, headache
Counselling points/notes	Inhaler is replaced weekly. Requires a challenge test with measures of lung function pre and post dose under supervision to ensure tolerability		

14.3.5 **Laxatives**

Chronic use of laxatives is often required and acute fecal impaction or distal intestinal obstructive syndrome (DIOS) can be the cause of an emergency admission to hospital (see Chapter 7). See Tables 14.46–14.50.

Table 14.46 Bisacodyl

Stimulant

Adult dose:	Paediatric dose:	Dosing in renal and hepatic impairment	Side effects
5–20 mg once daily, adjusted according to response	Oral 4 – 18 years, 5–20 mg once daily, adjusted according to response	Renal: no dose adjustment required Hepatic: no dose adjustment required	Abdominal cramping, nausea and vomiting, diarrhoea
Cautions and contra-indications	Avoid in intestinal obstruction, acute abdominal conditions, acute inflammatory bowel disease, severe dehydration		
Counselling points	Prolonged use can lead to electrolyte disturbances		

Table 14.47 Docusate

Probably a softener and stimulant

Adult dose:	Paediatric dose:	Dosing in renal and hepatic impairment	Side effects
Oral Up to 500 mg daily in divided doses, adjusted according to response	Oral 6 months–2 years 12.5 mg TDS (paediatric oral solution), 2–12 years 12.5–25 mg TDS (paediatric oral solution), 12–18 years up to 500 mg daily in divided doses, all doses adjusted according to response	Renal: no dose adjustment required Hepatic: no dose adjustment required	Abdominal cramping, nausea, and vomiting, diarrhoea
Cautions and contra-indications	Avoid in intestinal obstruction		
Counselling points	Capsules only licensed 12 years and above		

Table 14.48 Gastrografin®

Bowel cleanser (diatrizoate), used in meconium ileus distal intestinal obstructive disorder (DIOS) (unlicensed)

Adult dose:	Paediatric dose:	Dosing in renal and hepatic impairment	Side effects
Oral 20 ml up to QDS (unlicensed) Rectally 100 ml as a single dose	Uncomplicated meconium ileus, Oral Neonate 15–30 ml as a single dose DIOS (unlicensed), 1 month–2 years 15–30 ml orally as a single dose, 15–25 kg 20 ml as a single dose, >25 kg 50 ml as a single dose or <7 years 50 ml orally or rectally as a single dose >7 years 100 ml oral or rectally as a single dose	Renal: no dose adjustment required Hepatic: no dose adjustment required	Diarrhoea, nausea, and vomiting, intestinal cramping, intestinal perforation
Cautions and contra-indications	Asthma, hypersensitivity to iodine, hyperthyroidism		
Counselling points	Intravenous prehydration is essential in neonates and infants. Fluid intake should be encouraged for 3 hours after administration. *By mouth*, for child bodyweight under 25 kg, dilute *Gastrografin*® with 3 times its volume of water or fruit juice; for child bodyweight over 25 kg, dilute *Gastrografin*® with twice its volume of water or fruit juice Unlicensed use in adults, dilute each dose with 10× its volume with water or fruit juice The risk of anaphylactoid reactions increased by concomitant administration of β-blockers		

Table 14.49 Macrogols

Osmotic laxative

Adult dose:	Paediatric dose:	Dosing in renal and hepatic impairment	Side effects
Oral 1–3 sachets daily, maintenance 1–2 sachets daily. 8 sachets can be reconstituted in a litre of water and drunk over 6 hours in fecal impaction	Oral Paediatric preparation: <1 year ½–1 sachet daily, 1–6 years 1 sachet daily, increased to 4 daily if required, 6–12 years 2 sachets daily, increased to 4 sachets daily if required > 12 years 1–3 sachets daily, maintenance 1–2 sachets daily. 8 sachets can be reconstituted in a litre of water and drunk over 6 hours in fecal impaction	Renal: no dose adjustment required Hepatic: no dose adjustment required	Abdominal discension, pain, nausea, flatulence
Cautions and contra-indications	Cautions: Cardiovascular impairment, renal impairment Contra-indicated: Intestinal perforation or obstruction, paralytic ileus, severe inflammatory conditions of the intestinal tract (such as Crohn's disease, ulcerative colitis, and toxic megacolon)		
Counselling points	Note availability of different preparations; standard and paediatric		

Table 14.50 Senna

Stimulant

Adult dose:	Paediatric dose:	Dosing in renal and hepatic impairment	Side effects
Oral 2–4 tablets (7.5mg) daily, usually at night	Oral 1 month–4 years 2.5–10 ml (7.5 mg/5 ml) OD, adjusted according to response, 4–18 years 2.5–20 ml, adjusted according to response	Renal: no dose adjustment required Hepatic: no dose adjustment required	Abdominal cramping, nausea and vomiting, diarrhoea
Cautions and contra-indications	Avoid in intestinal obstruction		
Counselling points	Liquid preparation only licensed 2 years and above, tablet preparation only licensed 6 years and above		

14.3.6 Liver

Medicines used for the management of CF-related liver disease. See Table 14.51.

Table 14.51 Ursodeoxycholic acid

Prevention of CF related liver disease in patients with evidence of liver damage due to inhibition of bile flow

Adult dose:	Paediatric dose:	Dosing in renal and hepatic impairment	Side effects
Oral Varying doses recommended, but 10 mg/kg BD commonly used	Oral 1 month – 18 years 10 – 15 mg/kg BD	Renal: no dose adjustment required Hepatic: no dose adjustment required	GI disturbances, gallstone calcification, urticaria, pruritus
Cautions and contra-indications	Do not use with radio-opaque gall stones, inflammatory diseases of the small intestine		
Counselling points	None		

14.3.7 Pancreatic supplements

See Table 14.52.

Table 14.52 Pancreatin		
Pancreatic enzyme replacement therapy in patients with pancreatic insufficiency		
Paediatric and adult dose:	**Dosing in renal and hepatic impairment**	**Side effects**
Variable, dependent on individual and fat content of meal. Dietitians advise patients on suitable regimen. The daily dose should not usually exceed 10 000 units of lipase per kg body-weight	Renal: no dose adjustment required Hepatic: no dose adjustment required	Can cause irritation to the mouth if retained in the mouth. Excessive doses can cause irritation to the perianal region
Counselling points	Take with a meal or directly after. The high-strength pancreatin preparations Nutrizym 22® and Pancrease HL® have been associated with the development of large bowel strictures, therefore their use is not advised in children 15 years or younger	
Available preparations	Creon® 10000, 25000, 40000, Pancrex, Pancrex V, Nutrizyme 22®, Pancrease HL®	

Fat soluble vitamins

The vitamins A , D, E, and K are fat-soluble and patients may need supplementation. There are a range of unlicensed food supplements that are commonly used. Licensed medicines should be used where possible.

14.3.8 Others

See Table 14.53.

Table 14.53 Ivacaftor (brand name: Kalydeco®)			
For *G551D* mutation in the *CFTR* gene			
Adult dose:	**Paediatric dose:**	**Dosing in renal and hepatic impairment**	**Side effects**
Oral 150 mg BD	Oral 6 years–18 years 150 mg BD	Renal: caution recommended if eGFR <30 ml/min (no dose reduction specified) Hepatic: avoid in severe impairment, unless benefit outweighs risk, in which case reduce dose to 150 mg on alternate days	GI disturbances, dizziness, rash
Cautions and contra-indications	Contra-indicated in hypersensitivity to any excipient		
Counselling points	Reference should be made to national funding arrangements before prescribing. Has many interactions with other medicines		

14.4 **Allergies**

Allergies to antibiotics are common in CF due to the high doses and repeated courses employed. Allergies within the CF population occur most commonly with β-lactams (in particular, piperacillin), although this finding may be as a result of their popularity as first-line antibiotic choices. Allergies to antibiotics have the potential to cause serious immediate harm (e.g. anaphylaxis), but those which preclude the use of certain antibiotics also limit treatment options to second-line antibiotics which may be less effective or more toxic. Exacerbations may take longer to resolve, requiring longer inpatient stays, and clinical outcomes may be poorer as a result. Treatment can also be complicated by anxiety in patients with previous experiences of allergic reactions leading to refusal of certain antibiotics.

Allergies range from type 1 IgE-mediated immediate reactions (e.g. anaphylaxis) to type 4 T-cell mediated delayed reactions (e.g. rashes with delayed onset). Identifying the type of allergy can help decide whether the antibiotic may be used again or not following desensitization.

Key points

- Allergies must be clearly documented in patients' notes
- Patients on courses of home IV antibiotics should be provided with and shown how to use an adrenaline pen
- Patients should receive the first dose of their home IV antibiotics in the outpatient clinic

14.5 **Desensitizations**

Desensitization to an antibiotic may be attempted in certain situations to enable use of an antibiotic to which the patient has previously reacted. Desensitizations are suitable for type 1 allergies where reactions occur as a result of mast cell degranulation. Mast cell degranulation occurs when sufficient quantities of allergen-IgE complexes bind to receptors on the cell surface causing cell breakdown and a release of a potent chemical mix of histamine, cytokines, and prostaglandins. These chemical signals result in swelling, itching, and in serious cases, anaphylaxis.

Desensitizations consist of 7 consecutive doses of an IV antibiotic which are given in succession with each dose increasing in concentration tenfold up to a final dose of the full concentration. It is thought that a gradual exposure of allergen-IgE complexes to the mast cell prevents deregulation and provides a temporary state of resistance to allergy.

For example:

Ceftazidime 2g desensitization schedule

Ceftazidime 0.002 mg in 100 ml sodium chloride 0.9% over 30 mins, followed by:

Ceftazidime 0.02 mg in 100 ml sodium chloride 0.9% over 30 mins, followed by:

Ceftazidime 0.2 mg in 100 ml sodium chloride 0.9% over 30 mins, followed by:

Ceftazidime 2 mg in 100 ml sodium chloride 0.9% over 30 mins, followed by:

Ceftazidime 20 mg in 100 ml sodium chloride 0.9% over 30 mins, followed by:

Ceftazidime 200 mg in 100 ml sodium chloride 0.9% over 30 mins, followed by:

Ceftazidime 2000 mg in 100 ml sodium chloride 0.9% over 30 mins

Key points

- Desensitization attempts should only be made with Type 1 IgE-mediated immediate reactions (e.g. anaphylaxis)
- Desensitizations should only be administered to inpatients with a doctor present on the ward
- Resuscitation equipment should be at hand
- Subsequent treatment doses must be given as an infusion and no doses missed for the course
- Desensitizations need to be performed for each course prescribed and repeated if more than 1 dose omitted

References

Ashley C, Currie A, UK Renal Pharmacy Group. *The Renal Drug Handbook*, 3rd edn. Oxford: Radcliffe Publishing, 2009.

Cheng K, Ashby D, Smyth RL. Ursodeoxycholic acid for cystic fibrosis-related liver disease. *Cochrane Database Syst Rev* 2012;CD000222.

CF Trust Antibiotic Working Group. *Antibiotic treatment for cystic fibrosis*. CF Trust. May 2009.

CF Trust. *Pharmacy Standards in Cystic Fibrosis Care 2011*. CF Trust, 2011.

CF Trust. *Standards for the Clinical Care of Children and Adults with Cystic Fibrosis in the UK*, 2nd edn. CF Trust, 2011.

Joint Formulary Committee. *British National Formulary*, 65th edn. London: British Medical Association and Royal Pharmaceutical Society of Great Britain, 2013.

Paediatric Formulary Committee. *British National Formulary for Children 2013*. London: British Medical Association and the Royal Pharmaceutical Society of Great Britain, 2013.

Redfern J, Webb K. Benefits of a dedicated cystic fibrosis pharmacist. *J Royal Soc Med* 2004;97:2–8.

Useful internet resources

<http://www.cochrane.org>
Cochrane collaboration of systematic reviews, including a number specific to CF.

<http://www.cysticfibrosismedicine.com>
Protocols for the treatment and management of CF in adults and children, developed at the Leeds CF Centre.

<http://www.cfinfo.org>
UK site developed by CF health professionals, with information about parenthood for people with CF.

<http://www.ecfs.eu>
European Cystic Fibrosis Society, with links to useful guidelines (including standards of care) and consensus reports.

<http://www.cftrust.org.uk>
Website of the national UK CF charity. Contains information for patients and links to standards of care and consensus guidelines for management of CF.

<http://www.cff.org>
Patient-centred web forum of the US national CF charity.

<http://www.ecorn-cf.eu>
Europe-wide advice forum for patients, carers, and health professionals.

<http://www.cfgenetherapy.org.uk>
Website of the CF Trust-funded gene therapy research consortium, currently engaged in a multi-dose gene therapy trial (2014).

<http://www.uhs.nhs.uk/OurServices/Childhealth/TransitiontoadultcareReadySteadyGo/Transitiontoadultcare.aspx>
UK Tool to help prepare young people and families for transition (not CF-specific).

Index